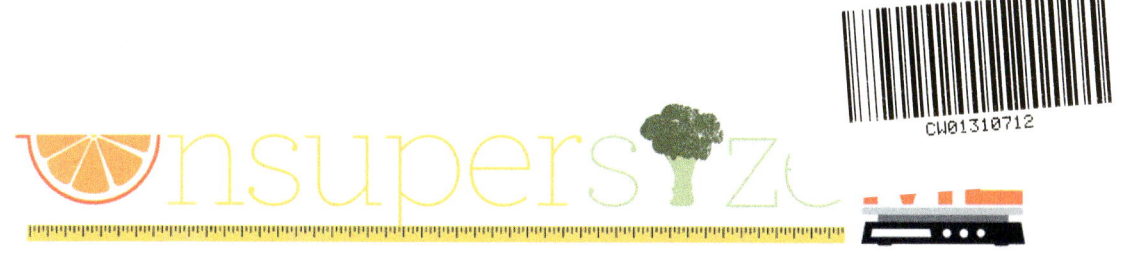

THE COOKBOOK

Carly Asse and Liz Smith

With special guest contributors

To all the staff + visitors at Dial House,

Please use and enjoy this cookbook, copy recipes, share them with your friends. This book was written to help people achieve better health in body and mind, so the more people enjoy it the better!

Yours in health,

Liz & Carly.

CONTENTS

Foreword 4

Introduction 5

About the Authors 6

Guest Contributors 8

Essential kitchen tools and techniques 9

Recipes 11

Brilliant breakfasts 12
    Breakfast oatmeal 13
    Breakfast super smoothie 15
    Power toast 16
    On-the-go breakfast power bars 18

Weekend breakfast and brunch 20
    Tofu scramble 21
    Buckwheat pancakes 22

Excellent entrées 24
    Corn chowder 25
    Roasted tomato and pesto pasta 27
    'Anything goes' vegetable curry 29
    Cuban black beans 32
    No'Chos 34
    Triple mushroom risotto 36
    Greek-style quinoa-stuffed peppers 38
    Grilled veggie pockets 40
    Roasted sweet potato and chickpea tagine 42
    Macaroni no-cheese 44
    Plant-based pizzas 46

Supercharged salads and sides 49
    Warm spinach, mushroom and potato salad 51
    Pink slaw with avocado 53
    Mushroom, lemon and coriander rice 54
    Chili garlic green beans 56
    Yucca fries 58
    Citrus salsa Fresca 59
    Perfect-every-time potato fries 60
    Fire roasted tomatoes 62

Dips and dressings to die for 63
- Hummus 64
- Holy guacamole 66
- Lemon tahini dressing 68
- *UnSupersize Us* signature dressing 70
- Balsamic vinaigrette 71

Delicious desserts and bakes 72
- Coconut chia pudding with mango 73
- Thai basil and lemongrass ice cream 75
- Mayan-spiced chocolate muffins with fudge frosting 77
- Sweet potato brownies with macadamia-vanilla cream 79
- Banana zucchini bread 81

Juices and mocktails 83
- Veggie power 84
- Mean green 86
- Florida special 88
- Cold buster 90
- Virgin mojito 91
- Non-alcoholic Piña Colada 93

Secret-weapon snacks 94
- Sundried tomatoes 95
- Tamari-roasted pumpkin seeds 96
- Chia berry jam 97
- Cherry-strawberry-chocolate smoothie 99
- Healthy cacao-date 'truffles' 100

More Resources 102

Foreword

By **Dr. Mohammad Ashori**

My name is Mohammad Ashori M.D. I did my medical school at UCLA and completed my residency in Family Medicine in 2009 at UCLA. I got a healthy serving of Western medicine during my training and appreciate the advances we have made in treating illnesses.

Our war on disease, however, hasn't been terribly successful. Though we would like to boast that as family doctors we are doing a lot of preventative medicine, the reality is that we're not. We test for diabetes and cholesterol and once the lab values meet the threshold for the disease, we pull out some medications from our arsenal to treat it.

But true prevention is empowering the patient, to inform them of what could potentially happen if they were to disregard their health. We disregard our health when we don't sleep enough, when we live with too much stress, don't get enough exercise, and eat what is marketed to us instead of what is actually good for us.

So what is good for us to eat? If you are having a tough time deciding, then here is a quick anecdote from one of my recent patients. He was obese, on medication for blood pressure and cholesterol, and needed insulin injections. With a plant based diet and some physical activity, he was able to lose some weight, but more significantly, he managed to come off his insulin and his cholesterol meds.

It's very tough for me to prescribe a healthy diet and exercise to my patients, because change is hard, but I assure you it has the least side effects compared to all the different medications that are out there. It's so easy to prevent hypertension, high cholesterol, and diabetes simply by eating a healthy diet. This book can show you how.

Are you interested in eating for better health but finding it hard to make the switch? It's okay, it's normal to find change hard - and I promise you, it will pass. Just try it and experiment with the recipes, and looking after your health will become a habit.

To your good health.

Dr. Mo

Introduction

UnSupersize Me – The Cookbook is a response to overwhelming demand -- demand from viewers, users of our online course, and supporters on social media - people who wanted to have the tools at home to eat the kind of healthy, whole food plant-based meals and snacks that helped Tracy lose 200lbs in a year and put the *UnSupersize Us* subjects back on the way to regaining optimal health in just six weeks

Our recipes are simple to create. They include tasty whole food plant-based versions of a few of the family favorite dishes that viewers wanted to see, such as mac n'cheese, breakfast pancakes, pizza and curry. They are full of flavor and draw inspiration from cuisines from all over the world to showcase the wonderful variety of food you can eat and enjoy on a whole food plant-based diet.

Before we get down to the business of cooking, we'd like to offer our thanks to our families and friends who have supported us and helped out with the making of this book in various ways, especially **Sandy Blaser Asse** for her recipes and help with the food photography; Carly's mom, **Marilyn Wall**, for always being ready to taste test, especially the desserts; all of our guest contributors for their ideas and input, our designers **Patrick Sanders** and **Simon Carter**, and our editor, **Lina Conlin**, for all her hard work. We love you all!

Enjoy cooking and enjoy your new healthy lifestyle!

Carly and Liz

About the Authors

Carly Asse

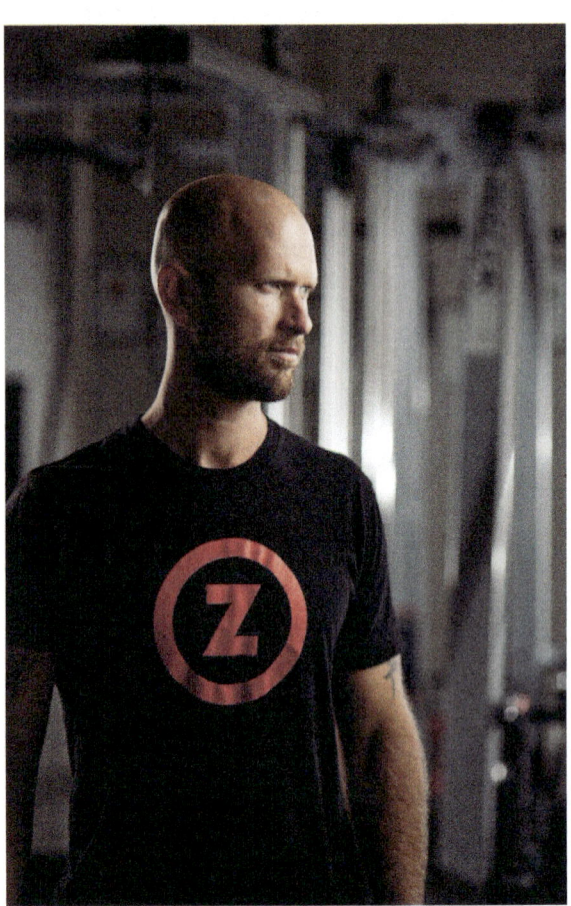

Carly has been a personal trainer and whole food plant-based nutrition expert for over 15 years. His approach of tailor-made exercise plans and a whole food plant-based diet has now helped hundreds of people transform their lives, including weight loss success stories of 100lbs and more, including of course Tracy Ryan, the subject of Carly's first health and weight loss documentary *UnSupersize Me*. Carly owns and trains at Zen Fitness in Gainesville, Florida, where his dedicated team helps people improve their bodies, lives and health.

Find Carly at http://unsupersizeme.com/

Liz Smith

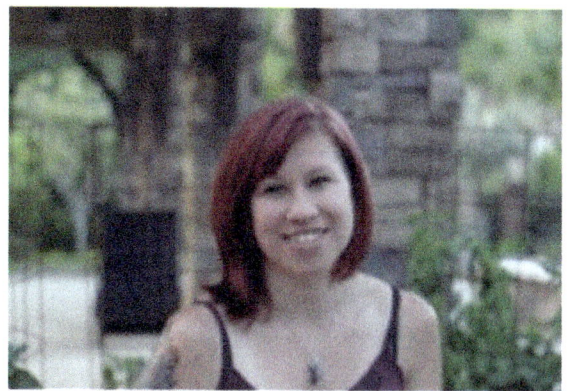

Liz is a food and health writer and editor from Leeds, UK. As well as writing the *UnSupersize Me* book and e-guide series, Liz was also one of the five subjects of Carly's second documentary, *UnSupersize Us*, so she has personal experience of how this approach can really make a difference to your health in a relatively short space of time. She is a passionate advocate of the *UnSupersize Me* approach for health and wellbeing as well as weight loss, particularly about the impact of nutrition and fitness on mental health.

Find Liz at http://wordsceneservices.co.uk

Guest Contributors

Sandy Blaser Asse has been on the whole food plant-based diet for several years, is widely known to be an excellent cook and has a wealth of knowledge about whole food plant-based cooking. She was a vital part of the *UnSupersize Us* support crew and provided many a delicious meal during filming. Sandy has provided several recipes for this book and was also indispensable during the recipe testing and photography phase.

Molly Patrick is a whole food plant-based nutrition coach currently based in Hawaii. Her website, Clean Food Dirty Girl, offers judgement-free health and nutrition coaching based on the whole food plant-based diet. Molly's mission is to help and empower people with the right tools and information to prevent disease and stay healthy for life.
Find Molly at http://cleanfooddirtygirl.com/

Molly Sexton teaches third grade in Gainesville and was one of the five UnSupersize Us subjects. Molly also won the plant-based Iron Chef competition, so her culinary skills are very well known and respected!

Steve Dent, a UK-based food blogger, creates original recipes on his blog, *The Circus Gardener's Kitchen*, often using fresh seasonal ingredients that he has grown himself. His aim is to show that vegetarian and vegan dishes can be exciting, nutritious and full of wonderful flavors and textures. Steve also writes about the politics of food, and what he regards as the looming unsustainability of many aspects of the food industry.
Find Steve at http://circusgardener.com

Essential kitchen tools and techniques

We'll be talking about a lot of different cooking techniques in this book and there are a few basic kitchen tools that we use a lot and that you'll need to make these recipes. Here are the essentials for your whole food plant-based kitchen.

A good set of sharp kitchen knives
Having a few good sharp knives is essential in a plant-based kitchen, because you'll be doing a lot of chopping! We recommend at least a high quality all-purpose chef's knife, a paring knife, and a serrated knife for chopping tricky tough-skinned customers like tomatoes. Keeping your knives sharp makes chopping a safer activity, so make sure you have a sharpener and use it regularly.

A high-speed, heavy duty blender
We use the blender a lot in this book. You'll need something that can cope not only with blending fruit and veggies for smoothies, but also tougher things like nuts and dried fruit. We recommend the Shark Ninja products, Vitamix or Nutribullet range.

A good quality heavy skillet (frying pan)
We sauté a lot (yes, it's a fancy word for shallow frying, but using a minimal amount of oil) and we find that for the best results, you need a good quality skillet. Cast iron and ceramic cookware is growing in popularity as concerns grow about the safety of non-stick coatings – we would always recommend you go as chemical free as possible for anything you're going to use for your food.

Food storage containers
Many of the dishes here will keep well for another day, or you might want to increase your quantities if you want to freeze leftovers for those days when you're too busy to cook. We strongly recommend you use glass or Pyrex for your food storage, or at the very least BPA-free plastic.

Juicer
We love juicing, and there is a whole section devoted to juice recipes and healthy drinks in here. Juicers start pretty cheap these days for the centrifuge-type juicers, but the cheaper ones are usually quite noisy and often not terribly efficient. Look at product reviews and comparisons for information about the best juicers within your price range. Some juicers can be quite bulky, which may be an issue in a small kitchen – if this is you, check out Philips' range of compact juicers that take up less space.

Grater/shredder
A few of our recipes also require the use of a grater/shredder. Either you could use an attachment on your food processor or pick up a manual one for a few dollars. Choose stainless steel instead of plastic.

Peeler
A sharp, comfortable to use peeler is another essential for veggies like potatoes and carrots. Having a good peeler makes short work of what can be a pretty monotonous task.

Stick blender
This is useful for blending up soups and soft fruit smoothies without having to go through the hassle of getting your food processor or heavy duty blender out (and clean it). These can be picked up at a very reasonable price online or in stores like Target and Walmart.

Baking sheets and pans
A large baking sheet is indispensable for roasting, which we do quite a lot of – many of our most popular dishes, like Carly's perfect-every-time potato fries and Sandy's yucca fries, are oven-roasted. You'll also need a few baking pans – a 1lb loaf tin and brownie pan will be helpful for some of these recipes.

Citrus juicer
You'll find that citrus flavors make their way into a lot of our dishes and drinks, so to get the most from your lemons and limes, you may want to invest in a citrus juicer. Manual ones come pretty cheap, but you can also get mechanical ones that save a little effort and extract more juice. If you don't have one, never fear – Liz has a technique for citrus juicing without any help. Simply halve your lemon or lime, stick a fork in the middle of the flesh, and squeeze it hard.

Recipes

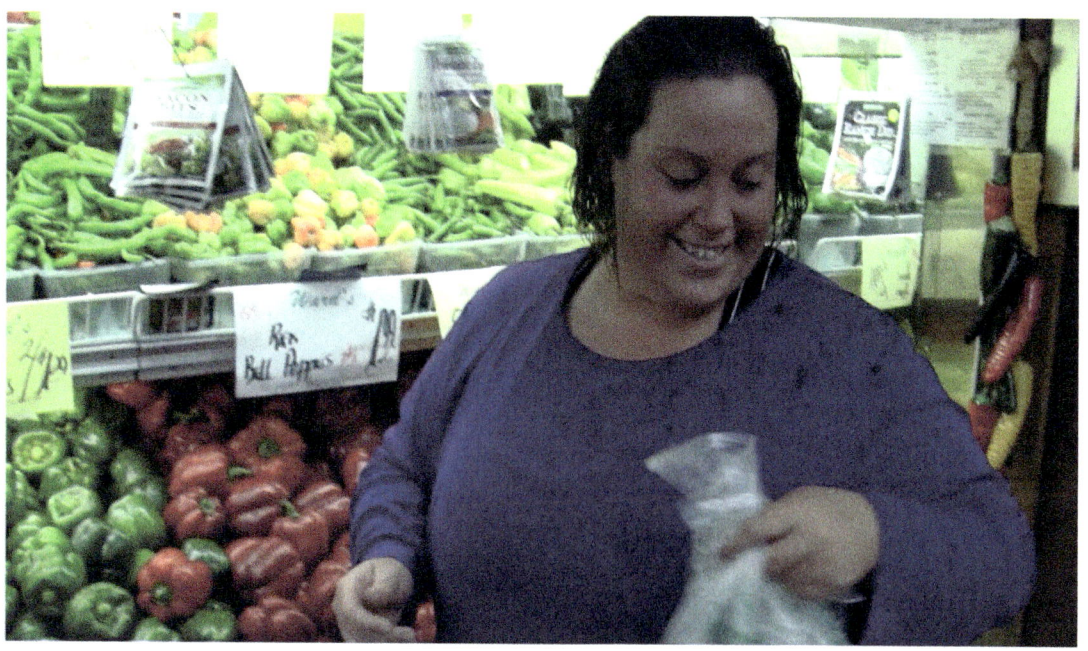

Tracy Ryan does her first whole food plant-based shop, as seen in UnSupersize Me

Brilliant breakfasts

Starting the day with a healthy breakfast is important. This is the main time when your body needs energy after several hours fasting while you sleep. Start the day without fueling your body properly and you risk an attack of the mid-morning munchies, which means you might reach for unhealthy snacks or be tempted by communal biscuits and treats at the office. Our healthy, quick and simple breakfast recipes will make sure you stay satisfied until lunch time. If you're really not an eat in the morning person, some of these can also be made ahead and taken with you to your workplace, school or for eating after your workout if you prefer to exercise first.

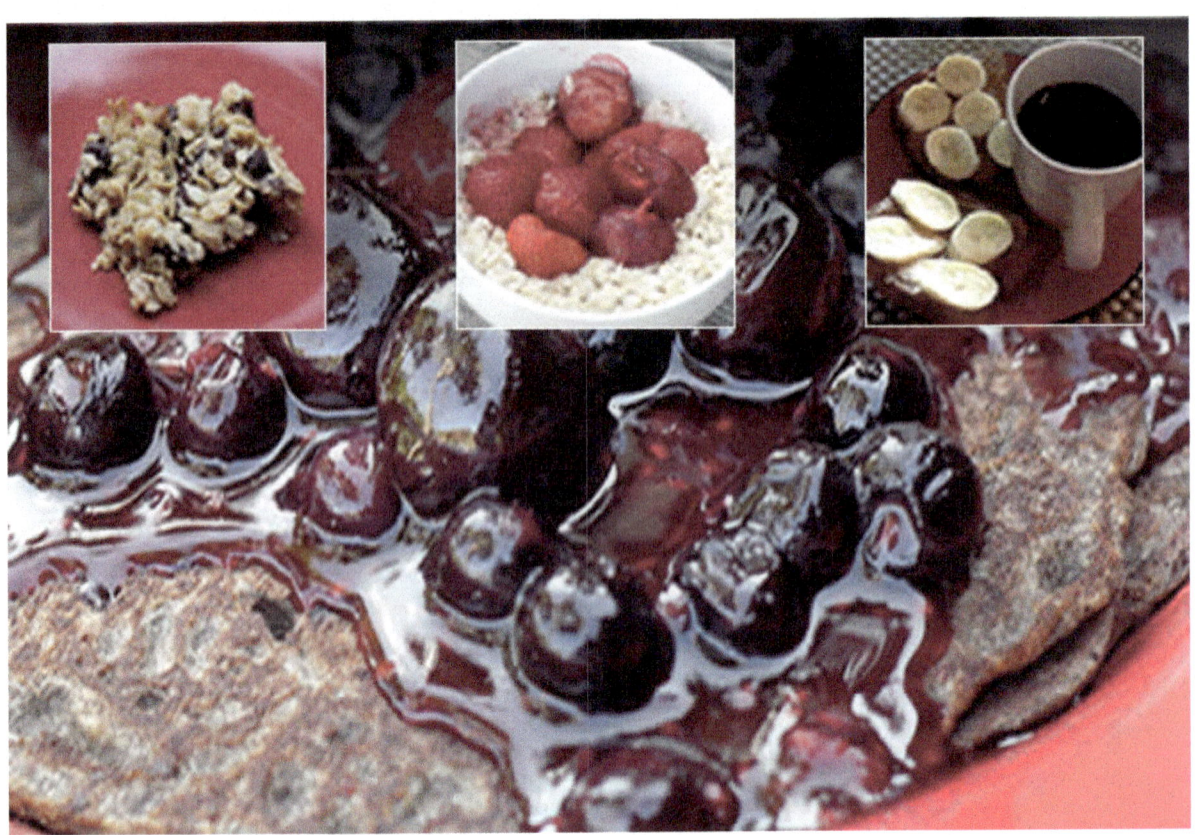

Breakfast oatmeal

Start your day like Carly does with slow-release carbohydrates and protein (yes, protein) from pure oats and an energy hit from fruit

Ingredients
Serves 1

- ½ cup oatmeal
- ¾ cup water
- ½ banana
- ¼ cup frozen berries of your choice

Make it

Mash up your banana with a fork – you can get it smooth or leave it a little chunky, depending how you like the texture of your oatmeal. Either way is OK, because you're still getting the plant-based goodness whether it's smooth or a bit chunky.

Add the oatmeal and water and stir to combine.

Microwave it

Microwave for 1 min 30 secs. Add berries. You can also add a little more water if you prefer your oatmeal a little thinner. Microwave for a further 1 min 30 secs.

Microwave tip: *Cover the bowl with a microwave-safe plate so the oatmeal doesn't boil over and you don't end up with a mess to clean up! Cleaning your microwave eats into your workout time…*

Don't have a microwave? Cook it on the stove

Heat until the mixture gets to boiling point, then turn down to a gentle simmer. Simmer for around 7 mins, then add the frozen berries and stir through. The berries should be defrosted and just starting to soften in around 3 mins.

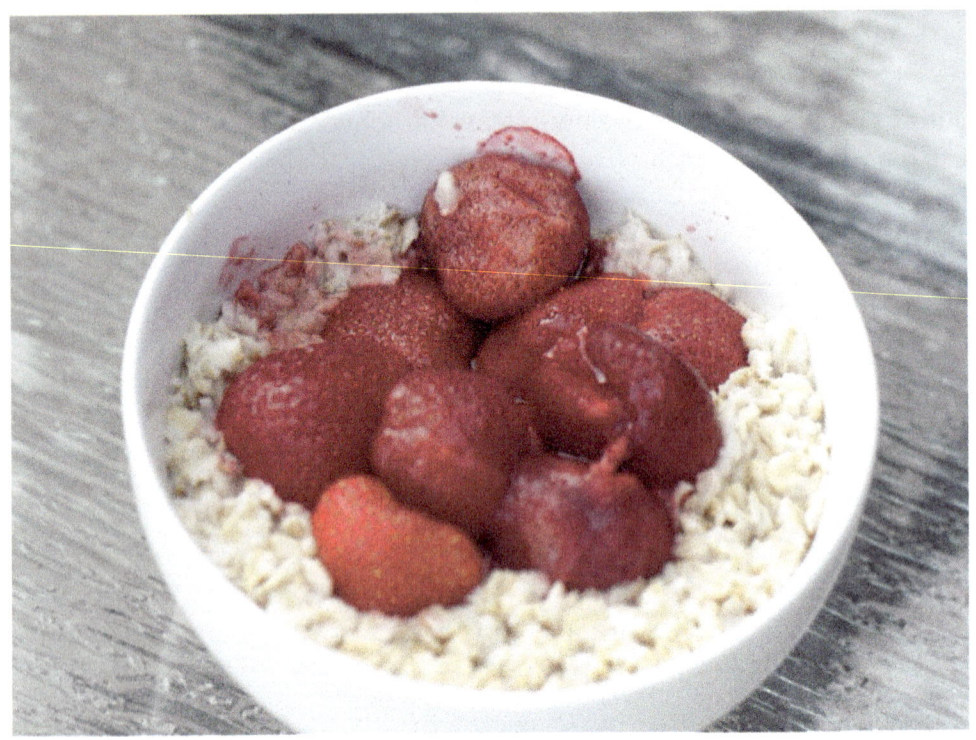

A note about oats

Oats are well-tolerated by most people, but some people with celiac disease cannot tolerate even gluten free oats. Oats contain a protein called avenin, which in some celiacs may provoke a similar reaction to gluten, most often causing digestive upset. Either brown rice or quinoa flakes could be used to make an oat-free version using exactly the same method. You can find these in health food stores or in the wholefoods section in the supermarket.

Variations

We don't want you getting bored with your breakfast, so here's a few ways to vary your oatmeal in the morning.

The protein hit – *stir through a spoonful of nut butter or add a sprinkle of raw nuts/seeds on top*

The energy boost - *Stir through some dried fruit, such as raisins or chopped dates*

The extra-creamy - *Make it with an unsweetened dairy free milk instead of water*

The Scot - *Add a pinch of sea salt*

Breakfast super smoothie

This supercharged smoothie makes enough for two hungry gym rats in the morning. Great for busy days when you don't have time to sit down.

Ingredients
Makes 1 smoothie

- 1 banana
- 6 dates
- Handful of fresh or frozen strawberries
- Handful of fresh or frozen blueberries
- 1 tbsp. flaxseed meal
- 2 cups dairy free milk of your choice (unsweetened)

Make it

Did we mention this is super easy to while also being healthy and full of good plant-based energy and antioxidants? Well, it is.

All you need to make this smoothie is a blender. You just throw the ingredients in, turn it to a high power setting, wait for all the ingredients to combine and pour into a glass or portable smoothie cup to go. Yes, that's really all you need to do.

Frozen berries may need a little more blending – when you think it's ready, turn the power off, give it a stir and check for any fruit chunks that haven't been blended and switch on again for a little bit if necessary.

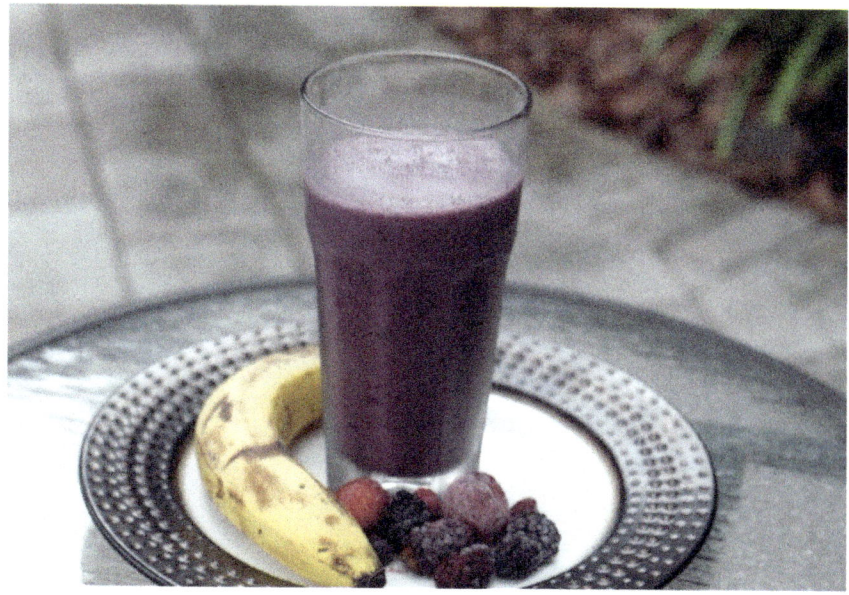

Power toast

If you're a morning workout person, you need to make sure you fuel those muscles and don't run out of steam halfway through, because that sucks – a body without enough energy doesn't perform well and doesn't get all the benefits. Remember, on a whole food plant-based diet, we're all about giving your body as much as it needs of all the good stuff, so forget all that stuff about carbs being 'bad' and nuts being too high in calories – because that's exactly what we *don't* worry about on a whole food plant-based diet. If you're exercising for 2 hours a day on the UnSupersize Me program, your body needs those carbs, because that's what it likes to use as fuel.

This power toast is ideal if you like to get your workouts in early – it's easy to make and can be eaten on the go, too.

Ingredients
Serves 1

2 slices sprouted grain bread (either whole wheat or gluten free - this should be from the freezer section in the store)
1 small banana
1-2 tbsp. almond butter
A little honey or agave (optional)

Make it

First, toast your bread. If using a toaster, you may need to put it through twice, as bread that's frozen will usually only defrost on the first cycle.

While the bread is toasting, peel and slice the banana.

Spread the toasted bread with the almond butter, then arrange the banana slices on top. Drizzle with a little honey or agave (it's easier if you use a squeezy bottle for this).

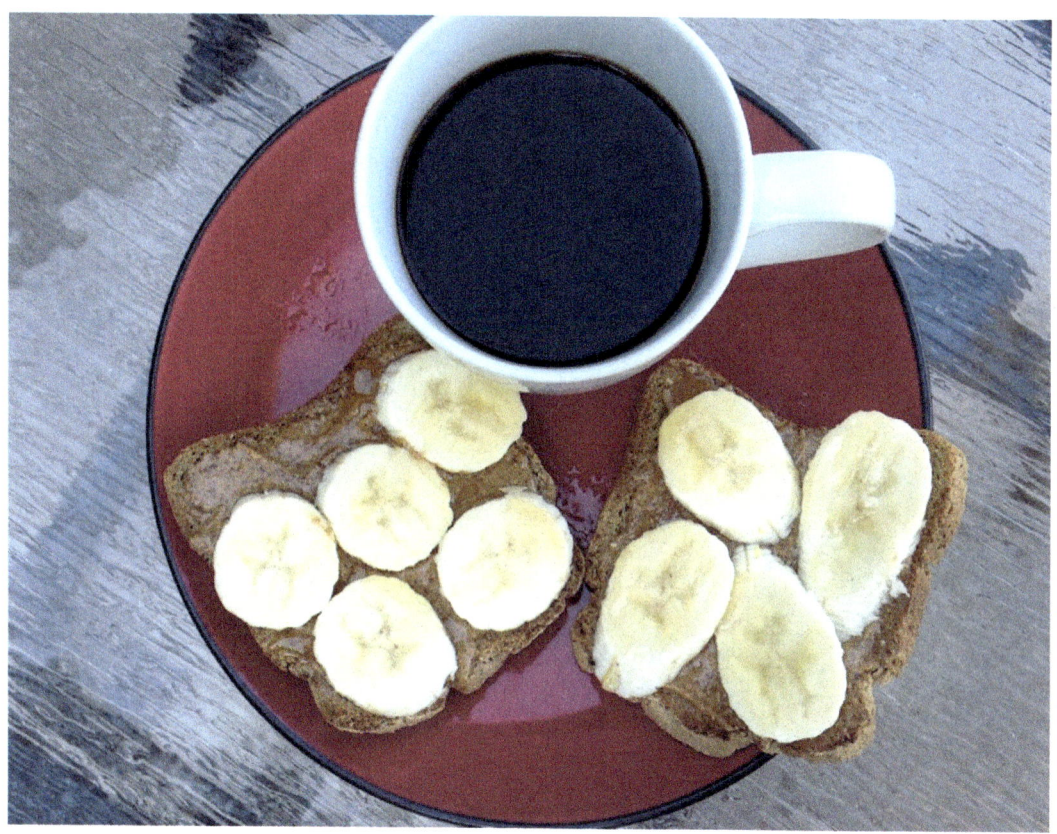

A note about bread

We only advocate either bread you make yourself from scratch from wholegrain flour or sprouted grain breads (like Ezekiel) that you find in the freezer section. Most breads that you find in the bakery sections of supermarkets or even bakeries these days are full of preservatives to make them last longer, as well as undesirable ingredients such as sugar, vegetable oils, gums and so-called "texture improvers", and even animal products like egg and milk. These are not whole food plant-based ingredients – we don't like chemicals in our food. Sprouted grains are also healthier, because the process of soaking and sprouting the grains breaks down some of the hard-to-digest proteins in the grains, minimizing the likelihood of digestive upsets and irritation.

If you're celiac or gluten intolerant, there are gluten free sprouted grain breads out there that you can buy online or in health/wholefood stores.

On-the-go breakfast power bars

These are a great portable food that's suitable for breakfast or a healthy snack. In the UK, these oaty squares are called flapjacks and will therefore be familiar to UK readers, but Liz found when she introduced them to the US crew they were quite a novelty!

Traditional versions of these usually contain butter and sugar, so these are a whole food plant-based version that's free of refined sugar and animal products and contain plenty of healthy seeds, nuts and a little sweetness from dried fruit.

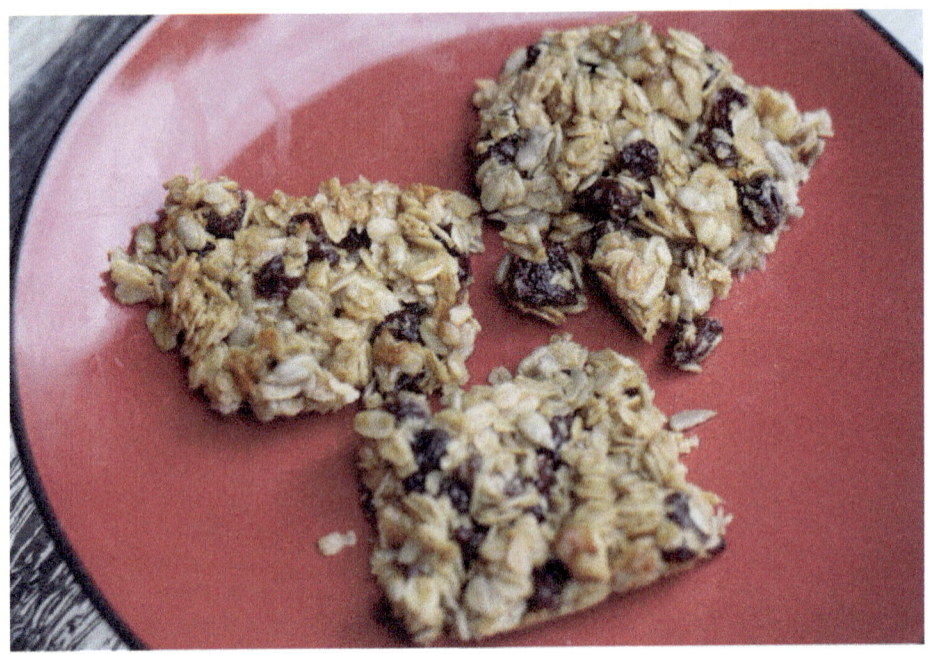

Ingredients
Makes 12 bars

2 cups rolled oats (use certified gluten free if required)
½ cup raisins (look for no added sugar or oil and sulphite free)
¼ cup pumpkin seeds
¼ cup chia seeds
½ cup pecans or walnuts, chopped
¼ cup natural sweetener (agave, maple syrup or date syrup)
2 tbsp. coconut oil, melted
pinch of sea salt

Make it

Preheat the oven to 350F/75C/Gas Mark 4

Line a baking pan with baking parchment

Mix all the dry ingredients together in a mixing bowl, then add the oil and sweetener and stir well to ensure everything is coated.

Pour into the baking pan. Spread the mixture evenly and then press down with a spatula, ensuring the mixture is compacted together.

Bake for 20-25 mins. It should be golden on top.

Allow to cool completely before cutting it into bars or squares. Depending on the sweetener used, the mixture can be a little crumbly, especially if it hasn't quite cooled enough. 15-20 mins in the fridge should fix that if it's crumbling too much when you're cutting it.

Store in an airtight container in a cool, dry place.

Weekend breakfast and brunch

We've included a couple of recipes here for making on weekend mornings when you might usually want something a bit different to the usual weekday "make it on the run" fare when you're on the way out of the door trying to get to work, school or the gym. These are healthier, plant-based versions of the usual crowd-pleasers for weekend family breakfasts and brunches that everyone will enjoy. We've tested these recipes on our friends and family who aren't whole food plant-based or vegan and we've never had a bad verdict yet.

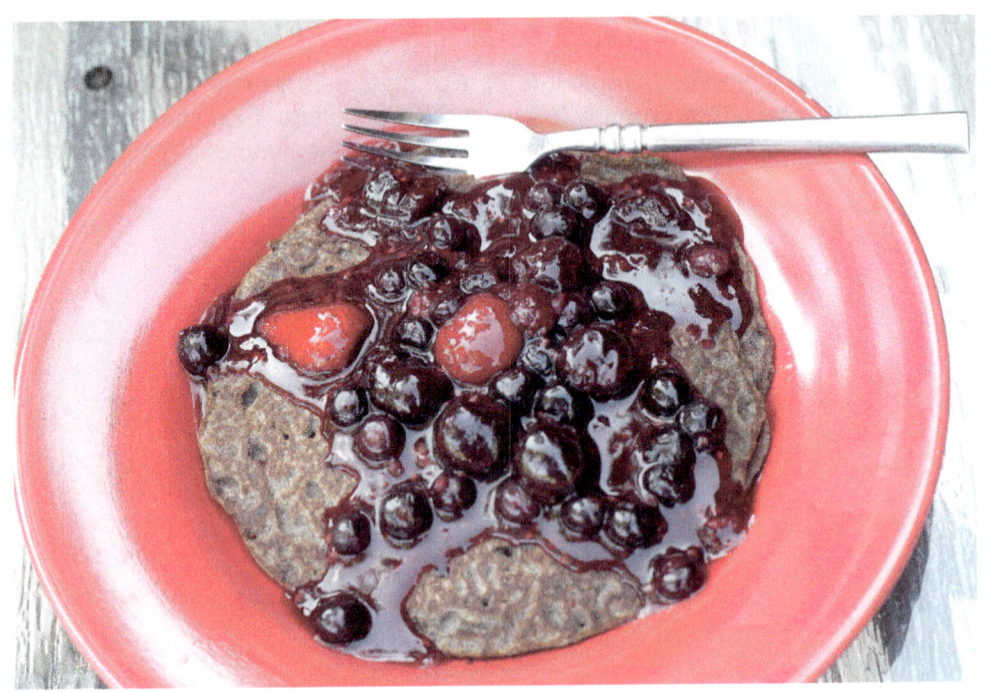

Tofu scramble

Who needs eggs when you can have this protein-packed breakfast using tofu? This tofu scramble is fully plant-based and includes kale and peppers for a healthy way to start your day. You can find firm tofu in most supermarkets.

Ingredients
Serves 2

1 pack firm tofu
1 bell pepper, any color you like
2-3 handfuls finely chopped kale
Olive oil, for stir-frying
½ tsp paprika
½ tsp chili powder
1 tsp liquid aminos
2 tbsp. nutritional yeast
Salt and pepper for seasoning

Make it

Finely chop the kale (unless using a ready-chopped pack). Dice the bell pepper.

Heat a little olive oil in a skillet.

Add the pepper first and stir fry for a few minutes. Drain the tofu, crumble it with your hands, and add to the pan, stirring in the same way as you would do when making scrambled eggs. You'll notice the texture is quite similar.

Stir fry the tofu for around 5 mins until it's heated through and combined with the peppers.

Add the kale and stir fry for 1-2 mins, then add the spices and liquid aminos and combine.

Turn the heat off and stir through nutritional yeast. Add salt and pepper to taste if required.

Serve with sprouted grain toast, or a side of grilled tomato or portabella mushroom. If you like more spice, you could drizzle over a little hot sauce!

Buckwheat pancakes

Pancakes are a weekend breakfast favorite, but traditional pancakes contain egg, milk and white flour, which we obviously don't recommend for optimum health. These plant-based and gluten free pancakes are a great alternative as an occasional weekend treat. The recipe is based on fiber-filled buckwheat flour. We serve these with a berry compote instead of syrup and butter.

Ingredients
Makes 6 pancakes

- 1 ½ cups buckwheat flour
- 2 flax 'eggs' (see below for how to make these)
- 1 mashed banana
- pinch of sea salt
- ½ tsp cinnamon
- ½ tsp nutmeg
- ½ tsp baking soda
- 3 cups dairy free milk of your choice (unsweetened)
- Up to 1tbsp coconut oil
- 2 cups frozen mixed berries
- 2 tbsp. maple syrup/agave

Make it

First make your flax eggs. For each flax egg, use 1 tbsp. flaxseed meal and 3 tbsp. cold water. Mix well and refrigerate for 15 mins. The flax eggs will take on a slightly gelatinous texture, which then plays a similar role to egg in baking.

Mix the flour with the salt, baking soda and spices in a mixing bowl.

Add banana and flax eggs, stir, then slowly start to add the dairy free milk, whisking as you go. If you don't have a hand whisk, you could just use a fork to do this.

Ensure the ingredients are all combined and there are no bits of dry flour floating on the surface, then leave the mixture to stand for 15-20 mins.

In the meantime, make the berry compote. Just add the frozen berries to a saucepan on a low heat, add the maple syrup/agave and 2 tbsp. water and simmer gently on a low heat. This takes around 10 mins – you want the berries to be defrosted, but there should still be some texture to them.

Add ½ tsp of the coconut oil to a shallow frying pan. The pan should be on a high heat to prevent the pancakes from sticking, so you want to heat it on max setting, but you may need to reduce the heat a little once they start cooking.

Once the oil is well heated (but it shouldn't be smoking), use a ladle to get enough mixture from the bowl for the first pancake. The ladle should be almost to full, but not overflowing. Coat the bottom of pan with the mixture and ensure it's evenly distributed.

The pancakes should take roughly 1.5 mins per side. If you feel like they're starting to overcook, turn the heat down a little.

Repeat this process for each pancake, adding a little coconut oil each time before you add the liquid to the pan.

Serve pancakes drizzled with the berry compote and a little maple syrup, if you want a bit of extra sweetness. But go easy on it!

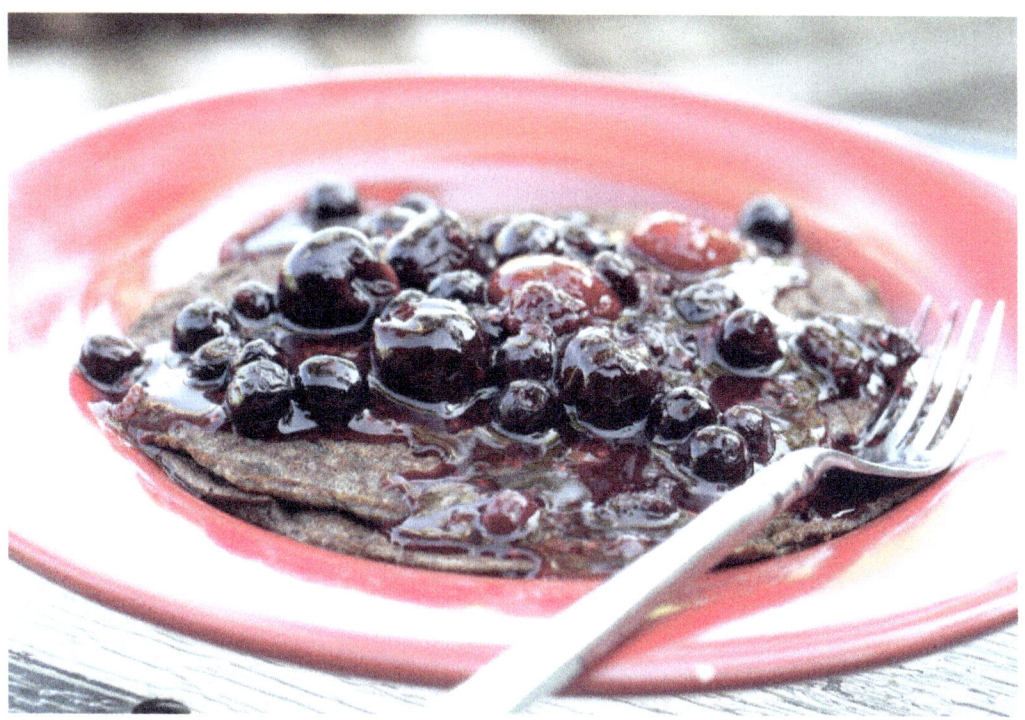

A note about buckwheat
Buckwheat is actually what we call a 'pseudo-grain' – it's actually a seed. It has a pleasant, nutty flavor and like quinoa, also contains some protein, so it will help you to answer all those "where do you get your protein" questions. Despite having 'wheat' in the name, it's actually gluten free, so it's safe for celiacs.

Excellent entrées

A selection of main dishes, from simple soups and pasta to hearty whole food plant-based adaptations of your favorite dishes from around the world. Your dinner table will soon become the place everyone wants to be.

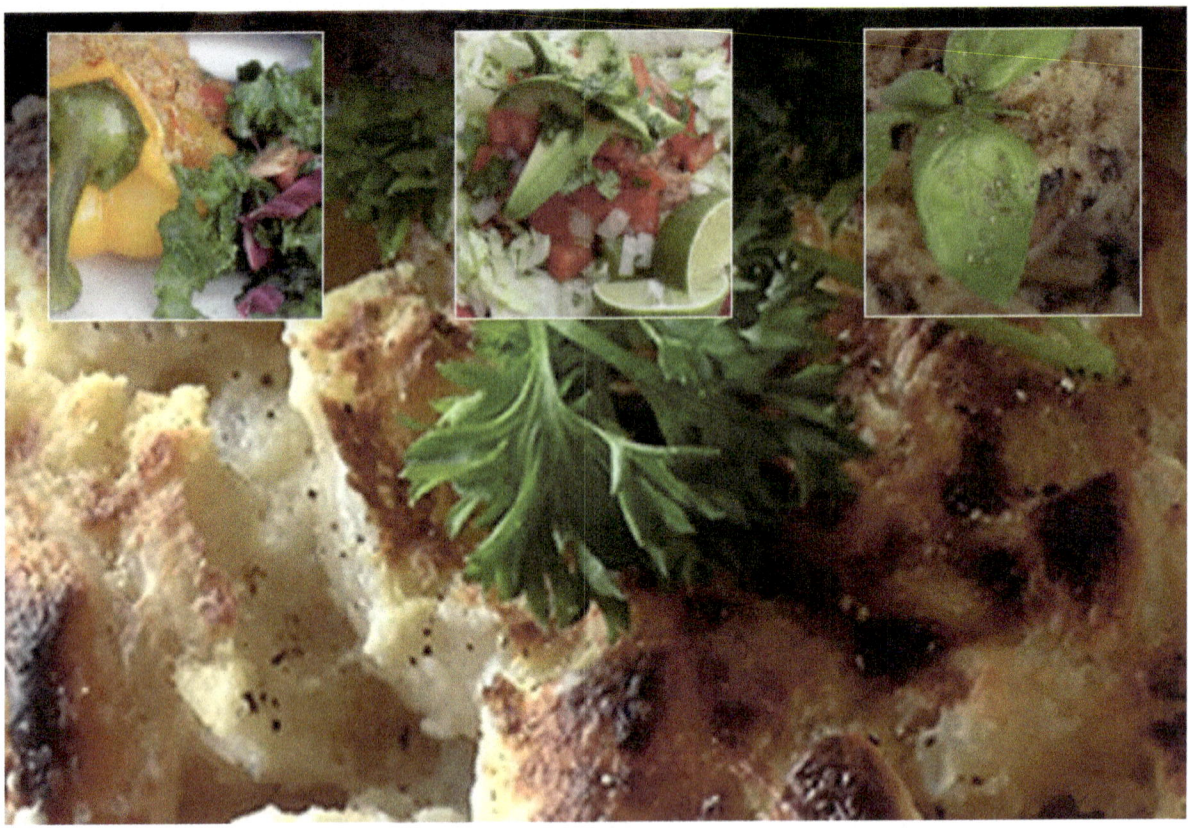

Corn chowder

Chowder is an American classic, but usually contains dairy and seafood. This version uses potato and cauliflower to get the classic chowder texture. It's more than just a soup, as anyone who's ever tried one of guest contributor Sandy Blaser Asse's most popular recipes will confirm. It's a little work to get the corn off the husks, but it's totally worth it, because this is the soup of champions.

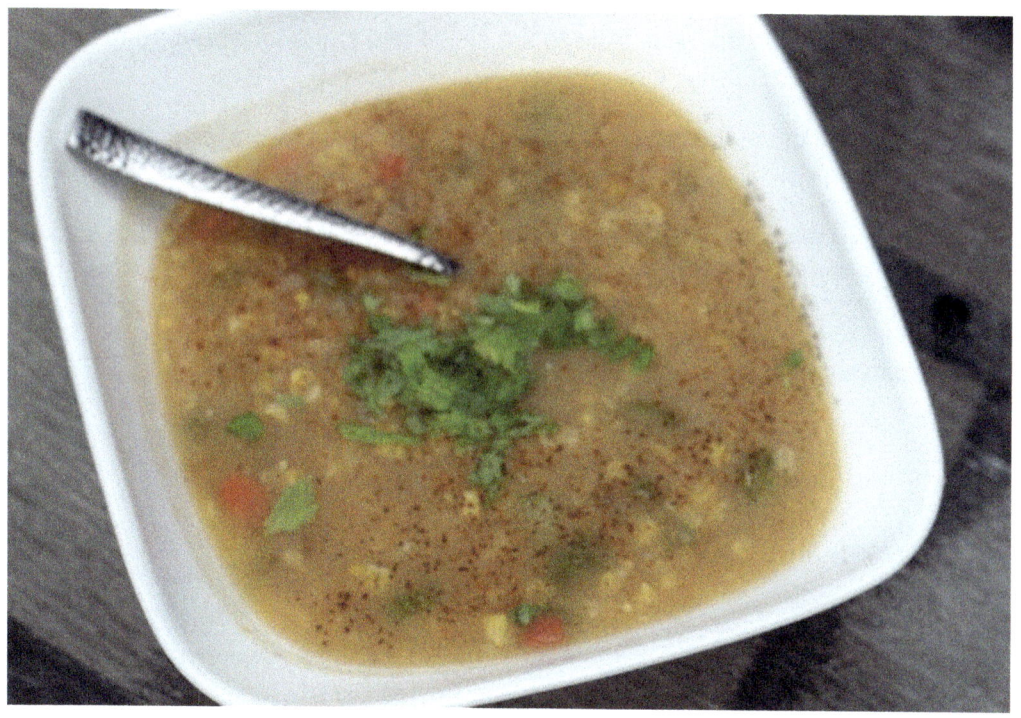

Ingredients
Serves 6

6-8 potatoes
1 head cauliflower
1 onion
4-5 carrots
4-5 celery stalks
2-3 garlic cloves
12 ears of corn on the cob
1 liter vegetable broth (stock)
Olive oil
Salt and pepper to taste
Flat-leaf parsley, for garnish

Make it

Peel and cube the potatoes, peel and slice the carrots, and cut the cauliflower into bite-sized pieces.

Boil the vegetables in the vegetable broth for around 15 mins.

Heat the olive oil in a skillet. Finely dice the onion and celery and sauté for a few minutes until translucent. Crush the garlic, add and sauté for a couple more minutes.

Meanwhile, cut the corn off the cobs. Add to the skillet and sauté for about 10 mins on medium heat.

Use a stick blender to blend the broth containing the potatoes, carrots, and cauliflower into a smooth, creamy soup.

Add the veggie from the skillet into the blended soup. Stir well and then allow to cook on medium heat for around 5 more minutes. Add salt and pepper to taste.

Serve piping hot – you could season with extra cracked black pepper and some chopped fresh flat-leaf parsley or even a little crushed chili if you like.

Roasted tomato and pesto pasta

Sandy's simple pasta recipe makes an easy, light meal for lunch or dinner. If you're gluten free, look for a brown rice or quinoa-based wholegrain gluten free pasta in the 'Free From' or Greenwise section of the grocery store instead of the whole wheat version. Watch for egg in the ingredients– stick to pasta that's just made from grains and water.

Ingredients
Serves 4

1 pack pure durum wheat (semolina) pasta (or gluten free equivalent)
4-5 medium tomatoes
½ Spanish/yellow onion
½ cup fresh peeled garlic cloves
¼ cup pine nuts
2 cups spinach leaves
A handful of fresh basil leaves
½ cup water
½ cup nutritional yeast
Olive oil, for roasting
salt

Make it

Turn your oven onto broil. Tightly pack garlic cloves in tinfoil with a few drops of olive oil and salt to start roasting the garlic.

Prepare the pasta in boiling water, according to package directions.

Core the tomatoes and cut the ½ onion into half again, leaving skin on.

Coat baking dish with a thin layer of olive oil, place the tomatoes and the two chunks of onion in and sprinkle with a little olive oil and salt.

Place baking dish in with the garlic – you should broil the tomatoes and the onion until charred on the outside.

Spread pine nuts out in the bottom of a skillet and heat on low to lightly toast them.

In a large food processor/blender, blend spinach, basil, water, ¼ cup olive oil. Blend well, then add pine nuts and nutritional yeast. blend again.

Finally take the charred skins off the tomatoes and the onion and add them to the blender, along with the roasted garlic. Blend until the sauce is an even liquid consistency. Add salt to taste.

Pour over cooked pasta and stir until the pasta is covered evenly.

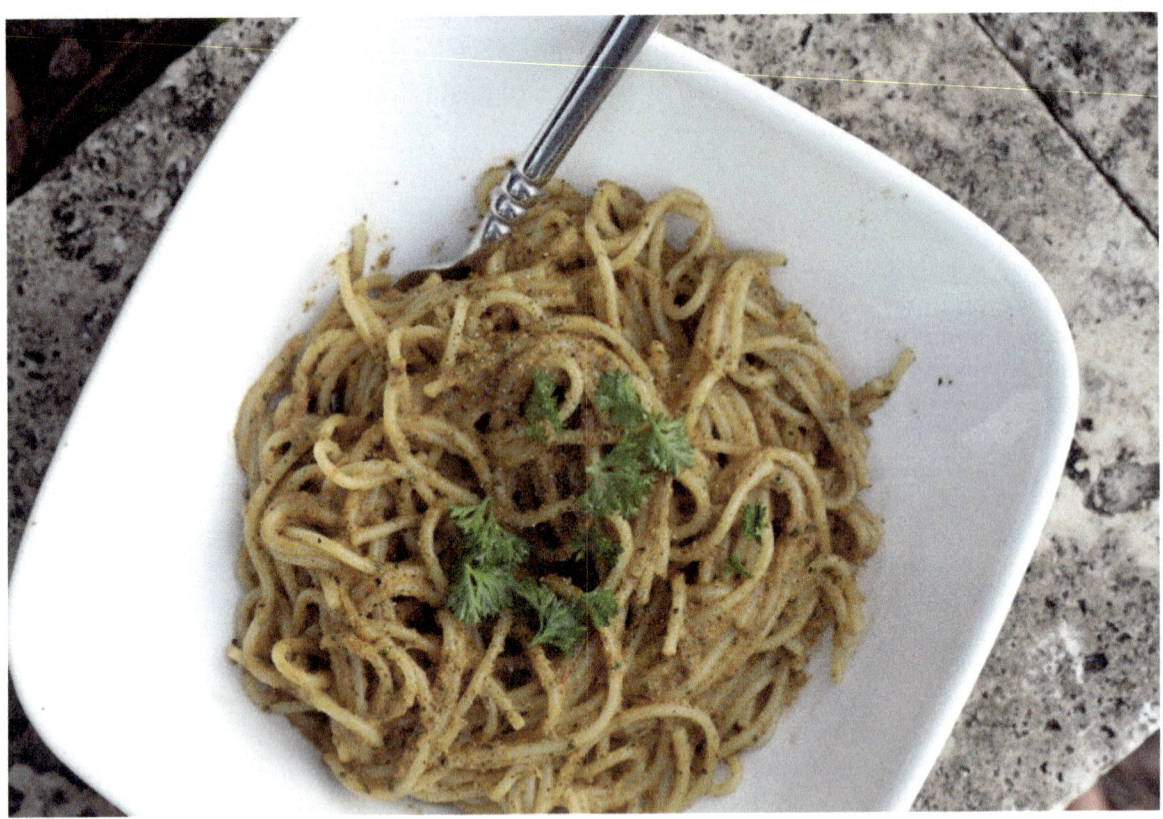

A note about nutritional yeast
Nutritional yeast is an excellent plant-based source of Vitamin B12, as well as being great for giving a savory, almost 'cheesy' flavor to your dishes. If you come across a dish you really like that's animal product-free except for the use of cheese, why not substitute some nutritional yeast so you get the flavor without the fat?

'Anything goes' vegetable curry

Curry is about as British these days as afternoon tea and Yorkshire puddings. The good news is that you don't have to do without curry on a whole food plant-based diet. This curry takes inspiration from the flavors of the Gujarat region of India, which is known for its vegetarian and vegan cuisine. You can use just about any vegetables you have in this, which makes it great for making use of whatever is in your veggie drawer that needs to be used quickly. Your own paste will taste better than shop bought, it's healthier, and it works out cheaper in the end too, once you've got all your spices. Spices can be bought much cheaper from ethnic food stores or markets and generally in bigger quantities so you don't have to keep replacing them.

Curry paste
Makes enough for curry for 4, but increase the quantities if you want to have some to use later – it will keep in the fridge in a sterilized jar or airtight container

2 tsp ground cumin
2 tsp ground coriander
1 tsp garam masala
1 tsp curry leaves, ground (either in pestle and mortar or grinder)
1 tsp turmeric
1 tsp cardamom seeds, crushed
1/2 tsp cinnamon
1 tsp chili powder (add more if you like more heat)
2 cloves garlic, crushed or minced
thumb-size piece of ginger, chopped and then crushed or minced
pinch of salt and black pepper
1 tbsp. coconut oil, melted

Make the paste

Dry roast the dry spices in a frying pan without any oil added first (takes about 2-4 mins) -- if you're in a hurry this isn't essential.

Combine all the dry spices and then mix in the garlic and ginger.

Add the coconut oil to get the curry paste consistency. Mix well.

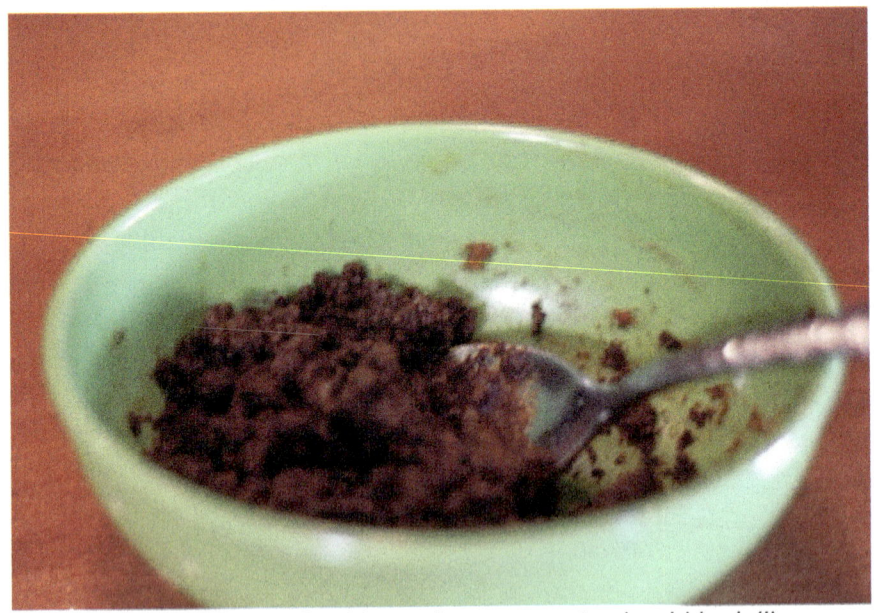
This is what your freshly made curry paste should look like

Make the curry

To make the curry itself, you'll need to fry some finely chopped onions in a little coconut oil as a base, because onions are great for imparting flavor.

Next, add your veggies in order of which ones take the longest to cook. You can use any veggies really – as a guide, you can base it on a root vegetable like potato, butternut squash or sweet potato, a legume like soaked green or yellow split peas (or chickpeas from a can if you want it to be ready quicker), followed by a variety of other chopped vegetables - eggplant works well in curry, as does zucchini or yellow squash, green beans, cauliflower, okra, peppers...anything goes! The important thing is to make sure that you use what needs to be used the most in your veggie drawer. That way, you'll avoid food waste.

Once all the vegetables combined in the pan, add your curry paste and a can of coconut milk, stir and combine well and leave to simmer.

If you use the split peas, it will take about 45 mins to cook, as long as they've been soaked, but of course that reduces if you use canned.

Serve with brown rice or with the mushroom and lemon rice side dish.

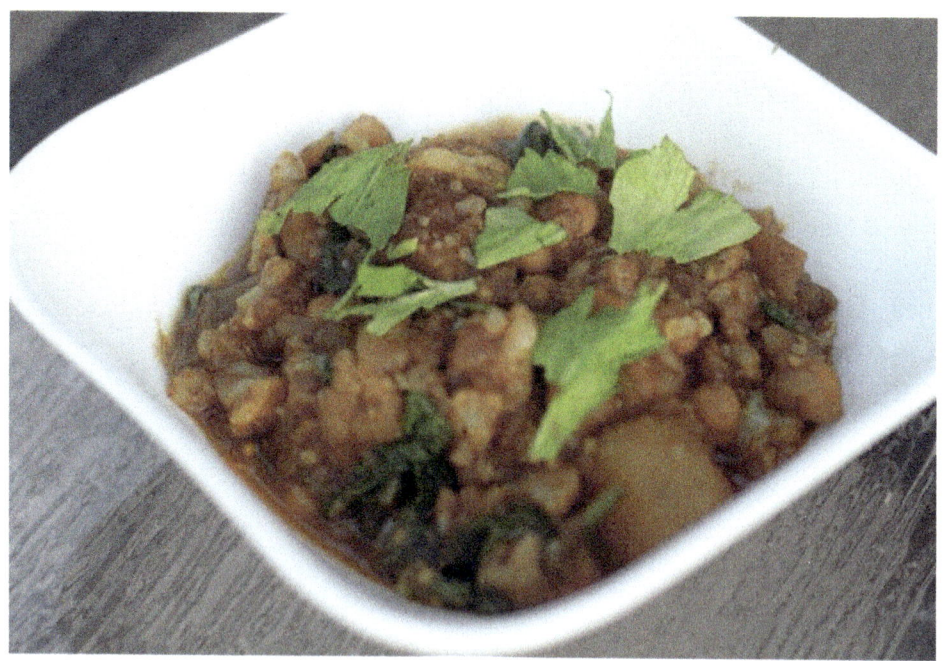

Why we love spices
Spices don't just give your food plenty of interesting flavor – they have health benefits too. Turmeric, for example, a root which gives food a yellow color and is often used in Indian cooking, is known for being anti-inflammatory and even anti-cancer. Garlic is anti-microbial, which means it helps fight bacteria. Ginger is known to alleviate nausea and be soothing to the gut, which makes it useful for travel sickness or morning sickness in pregnancy.

Cuban black beans

These traditional Cuban black beans are hearty, spicy and full of flavor. They are perfect served with yucca fries, as shown below.

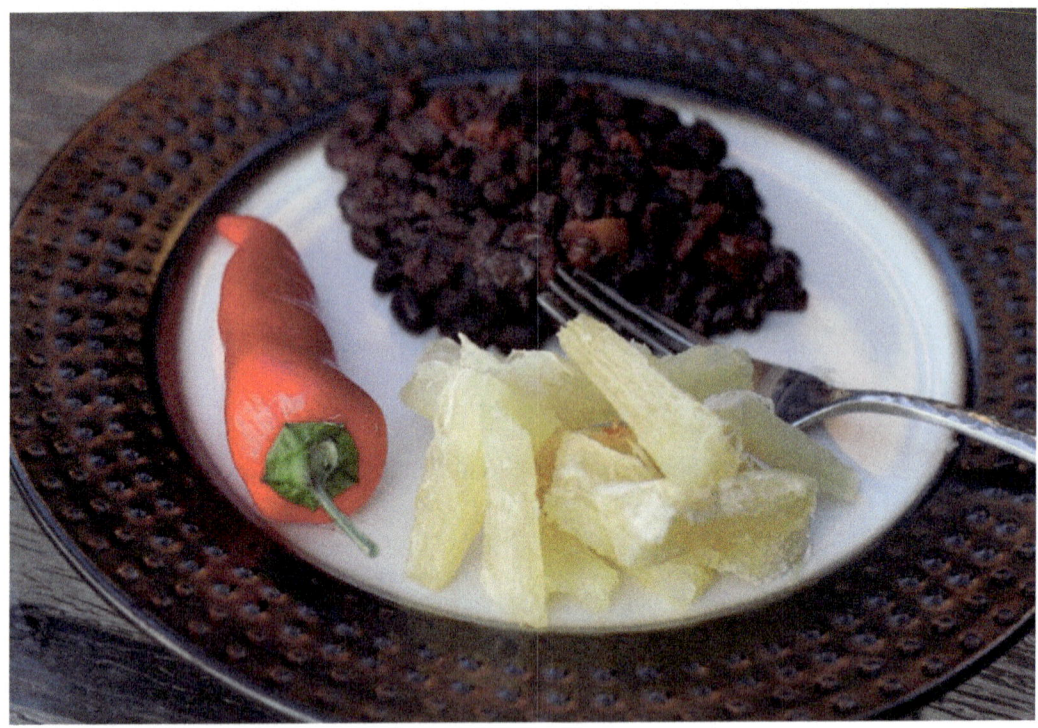

Ingredients
Serves 4

1 pound dried black beans, rinsed
10 cups water
1 tbsp. olive oil, plus extra for sautéing
1 yellow onion, diced
2 red bell peppers, diced
1 chili pepper, minced (optional)
4 cloves garlic, minced
2 bay leaves
2 tbsp. white vinegar

1 tablespoon ground cumin
1 teaspoon oregano
1 tablespoon sea salt

Make it

Soak the black beans for at least 4hrs (preferably overnight) in cold water. Drain and rinse when ready to use.

Add the beans to a large pot containing 10 cups of water and 1 tbsp. olive oil. Boil rapidly for 10 mins, then reduce to a simmer and cover. Simmer for around 50-60 mins until beans are tender.

In a skillet, heat a little olive oil and sauté the onion and peppers until translucent. Season with some salt.

Once the beans are cooked, add the chili, garlic, bay leaves, white vinegar, cumin and oregano and then the sautéed veggies. Stir and simmer on low to medium heat for around 15 mins, stirring occasionally to ensure it doesn't stick.

Serve hot with yucca fries or brown rice. Remove the bay leaves before serving.

No'Chos

Got a craving for nachos? Make UnSupersize Me star Molly Sexton's No'Chos instead. You'll still get all those Mexican flavors, but without the big bad dose of cheese or fried chips in unhealthy oil – and these are super quick to make for busy people. This uses canned refried beans, which are whole food plant-based friendly. You can also use ready-made salsa, as long as there is no added sugar on the ingredients list, or you can whip up your own using chopped tomatoes, onion, fresh chili and some lime juice. Add some jalapeños if you like it hot.

Ingredients
Serves 2

- 2 cups organic vegetarian refried beans (black or pinto)
- 4 cups shredded iceberg lettuce
- 1-2 ripe avocado, sliced (or alternatively make our guacamole recipe)
- Organic salsa
- Diced peppers, onions, olives- any raw veggie toppings you like
- Squeeze of lime

Make it

Heat up the refried beans for 1 minute in the microwave. Stir and heat for another minute (or heat for 4-5 min in a saucepan on low to medium heat).
Put shredded lettuce in a medium bowl.
Scoop beans and place in the middle of the lettuce.
Top with avocado, salsa and veggies and squeeze lime juice all over.
Enjoy!

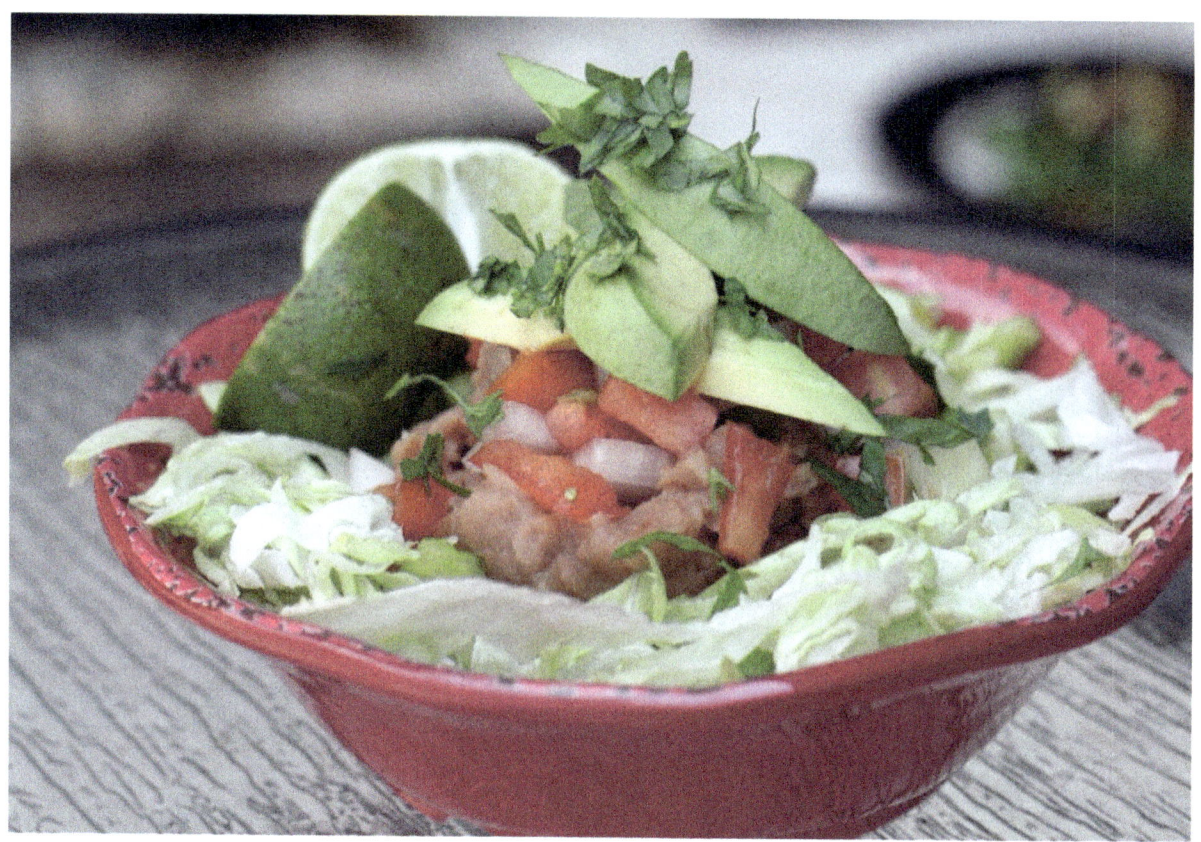

A note about avocado
Avocado is one of our favorite foods! It's full of healthy fats, which are important for your skin, brain function, and your heart, believe it or not – fat is not the enemy, you just have to choose wisely. Avocado is a perfect way to get your monounsaturated fats. We also permit the use of coconut and olive oil in small amounts. Choose your oils cold pressed if possible.

Triple mushroom risotto

Sandy's mushroom risotto is a tasty plant-based version of the traditional Italian favorite. This dish uses Arborio rice, which is a traditional Italian risotto rice. It is a white rice, but it's also very low-GI, meaning it's a slowly-absorbed carbohydrate that will fill you up for longer. Remember to stir your risotto frequently -- this is what will give you the creaminess without using any dairy. Serve with a green salad and *UnSupersize Us* signature dressing.

Ingredients
Serves 4
- 1 cup chopped trumpet or oyster mushrooms
- 1 cup sliced baby bella mushrooms
- 1 cup sliced shiitake mushrooms
- 2 cups Arborio risotto rice
- 2-3 cups mushroom broth (either from a mushroom bouillon cube or by simmering some dried mushrooms in water for around 45 mins and discarding the pieces)
- ½ cup dry white wine
- 1-2 tbsp. olive oil
- 2 tbsp. nutritional yeast
- Salt and pepper to taste

Make it
First, chop the mushrooms into small pieces. We've suggested some varieties to use for their flavor and texture, but you can use any variety you like.

Sauté the mushrooms in olive oil and salt to taste

Heat some more olive oil in another sauté pan. Add the rice and stir until coated with the oil on a low to medium heat.

Add white wine and stir until completely absorbed. Then start adding the mushroom broth – add enough to just cover the rice and keep stirring until it is completely absorbed. Repeat this process, adding a little mushroom broth at a time until it is absorbed. Don't let the rice stick to the pan – you have to keep watching it and stirring.

The rice is cooked when it is *al dente*, i.e. tender but still a little firm to the bite.

Remove the rice from the heat, then add the mushrooms, nutritional yeast, salt and pepper. Stir well. The rice should appear moist and creamy.

Serve immediately.

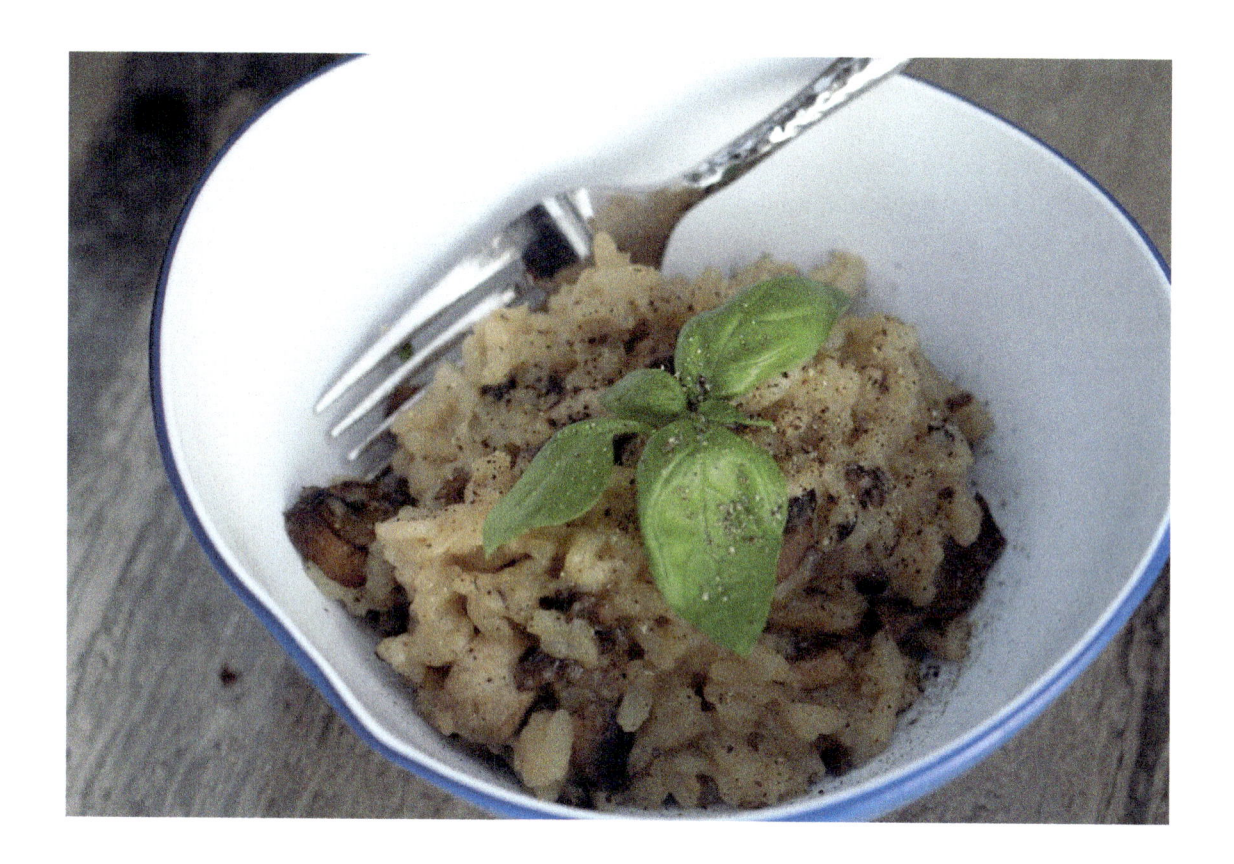

Mushrooms...a natural superfood

Mushrooms are a natural source of many of the minerals we need in our diets, including selenium, copper, magnesium, iron and phosphorus. The cell walls of mushrooms are indigestible unless cooked, however, so you'll get the most nutritional benefits from mushrooms if you cook them.

Greek-style quinoa-stuffed peppers

Bring the flavors of the sunny Mediterranean into your kitchen with these colorful peppers stuffed with quinoa, Kalamata olives, and veggies. These work well with a green salad and Molly Patrick's tahini lemon dressing.

Ingredients
Serves 4

4 whole peppers
2 cups quinoa
1 vegetable bouillon (stock) cube
20 Kalamata olives, stones removed and roughly chopped
1 onion, diced
2 large beef tomatoes, diced
2 cloves garlic, crushed
1 tsp dried oregano
1 tsp dried marjoram
1 tsp dried basil
2 tbsp. nutritional yeast
Juice of 1 lemon
Olive oil, for sautéing
Salt and pepper to taste

Make it
First, start cooking the quinoa. Add it to a pan of boiling water with the bouillon cube dissolved into it. Turn down to a simmer and leave for 15-20 mins, until the quinoa has softened but still firm to the bite. Drain and set aside.

While the quinoa is cooking, prepare the peppers. Cut them in half lengthways and remove all the seeds and white parts from the middle, so you are left with a shell for the quinoa mixture. Put them in a roasting pan and drizzle with olive oil, then set aside. Preheat the oven to 375F/200C/Gas 5.

Sauté the onions in a little olive oil until they are soft and translucent. Add the garlic, olives and diced tomatoes, stir and sauté for another 5-6 mins. Then add the herbs, lemon juice and nutritional yeast and stir to combine. Add salt and pepper to taste.

Combine the onion, olive and tomato mixture with the quinoa and then fill the peppers with it. They should be full, but not overflowing.

Roast the peppers in the oven for 25-30 mins. The quinoa mixture should brown slightly on top and go a little crunchy, which can give it some texture, but if you don't want this, cover the peppers with aluminum foil after 10 mins of roasting uncovered.

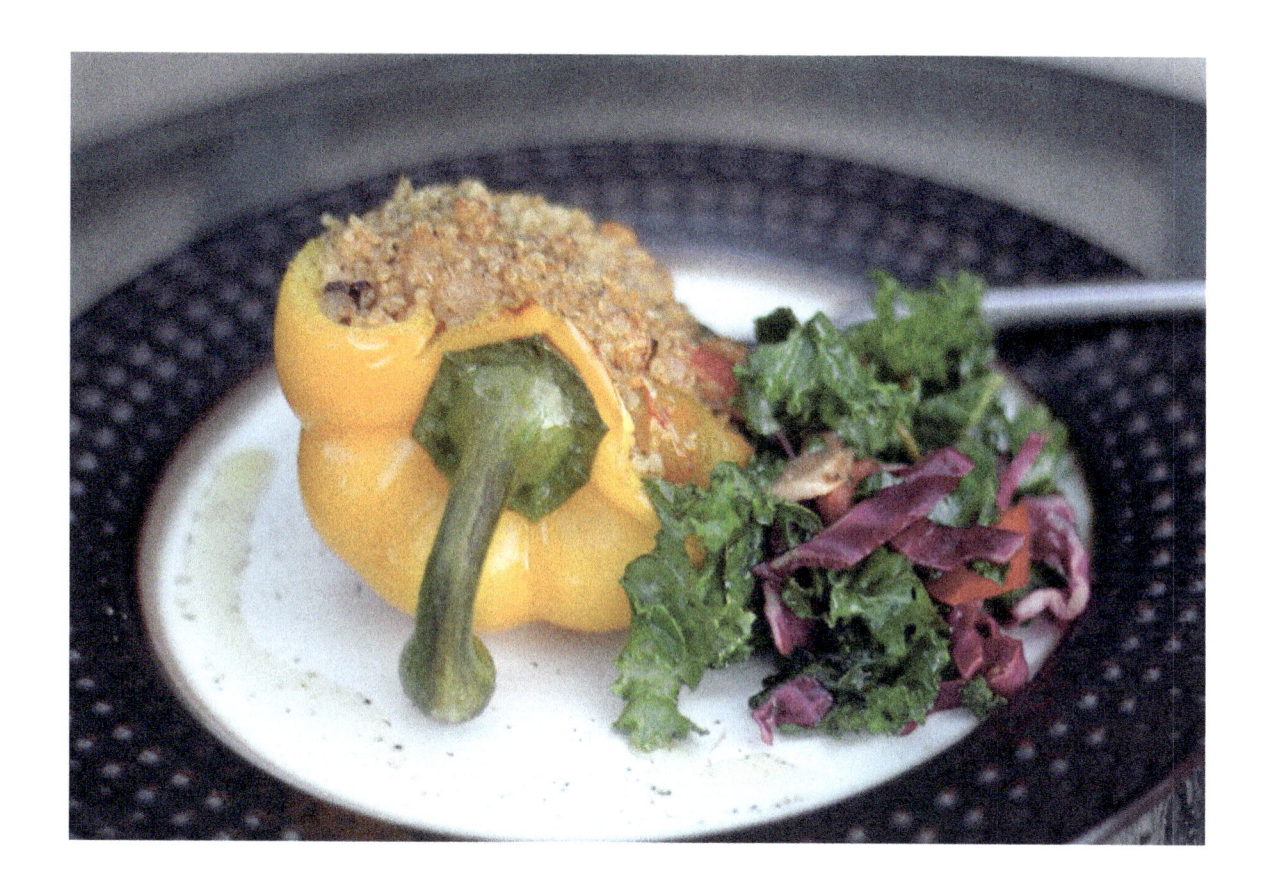

A note about quinoa
This gluten free 'pseudograin' (which means it behaves like a grain but it's actually a seed) is a really good source of protein. So now you know the answer when you're asked "but where do you get your protein"!

Grilled veggie pockets

Grilling isn't out of the question just because you're eating plant-based. These veggie pockets take a little preparation, but they're easy to cook on your grill and mean you'll always have something to make at a BBQ. They're easily portable too. Because they're cooked wrapped in foil, you don't have to worry about any cross-contamination with meat, fish or any allergens if you have food allergies. These are also great for fussy eaters because you can just include the veggies you like and skip the ones you don't.

Ingredients
Makes approx. 6 pockets

1 large onion
2 cloves garlic
4 sticks of celery
2 cups chopped mushrooms
4 tomatoes
½ head green or red cabbage
½ large eggplant
2 peppers
2 zucchini
2 yellow squash
6 medium potatoes
Olive oil
Liquid aminos
Salt and pepper
Chili flakes (if you like some spice)

Make it
Dice all the veggies finely and place them in separate bowls. Finely chop or crush the garlic and place it in with the onions.

Dice the potatoes and pre-cook them in the microwave on high for 10 mins.

Tear off 6 sheets of aluminum foil. The sheets should be big enough to wrap fully around a parcel the size of a small sub.

Add a little of each vegetable to the foil parcels in the proportions you want and then dress with a little olive oil, liquid aminos and a shake of salt and pepper. Add chili flakes if you like some spice.

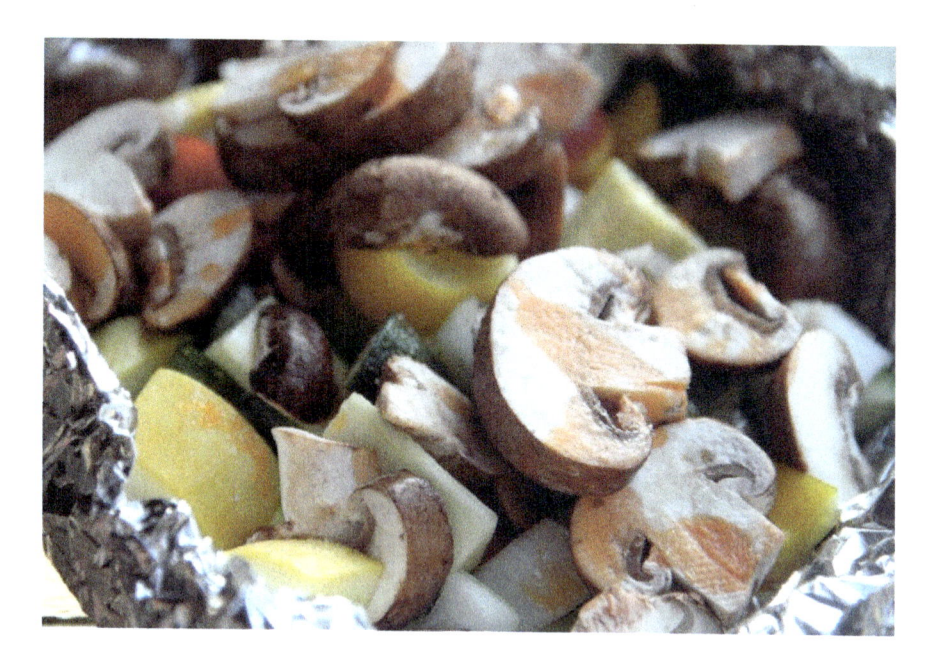

Place on the grill (BBQ) outside on a high heat for around 15-20 min. If you like your vegetables a little softer, leave the pockets for an extra 5 min. Be careful when removing them from the grill as the parcels will be very hot – use tongs to take them off and be careful of the hot steam when opening up the pockets.

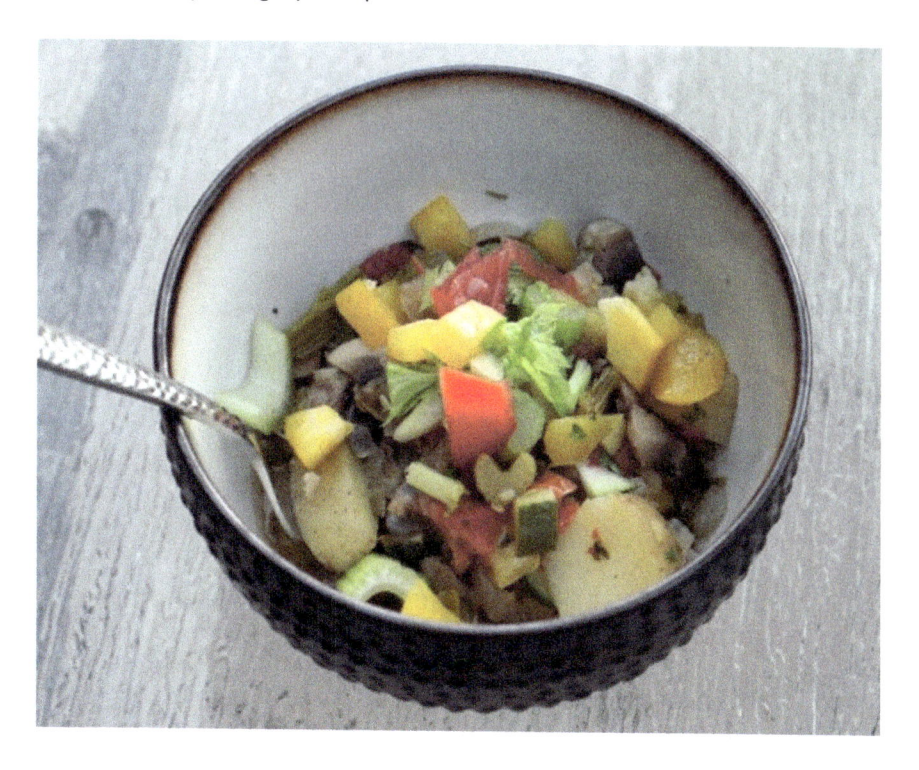

Roasted sweet potato and chickpea tagine

We're off to North Africa for this dish, which is full of fragrant spices and has dried apricots to add a touch of sweetness. This is a one-pot dish that's easy to make and great for a dinner party – the combinations of fragrant Moroccan style spices with sweet, sour and savory flavors in this dish will impress your guests.

Ingredients
Serves 6

3 medium to large sweet potatoes, peeled and diced
1 large onion, diced
1 zucchini, halved and cut into slices
1 yellow squash, halved and cut into slices
1 carrot, peeled and cut into slices
½ cup chopped semi-dry dates (such as Deglet Nour)
3 cloves garlic
Rind and juice of 1 lemon
½ cup chopped Peppadew peppers (or 1 thinly sliced fresh red chili pepper if you can't get your hands on these)
2 tsp ground cumin
2 tsp ground coriander
½ tsp cinnamon
1 tsp dried marjoram
1 tsp cayenne pepper
1 tsp agave/honey
2 tbsp. liquid aminos
2 tbsp. nutritional yeast
1 carton sieved tomatoes (passata)
2 cans chickpeas (garbanzos)
olive oil for sautéing
salt and pepper to taste

Make it

Preheat the oven to 400F/220C/Gas 6. Roughly chop the sweet potatoes into chunks.

Thinly coat the bottom of a roasting pan with olive oil. Once the oven is up to temperature, put the roasting pan in for around 2-3 mins to heat the oil up. Then add the chopped sweet potatoes to the oil, toss them to coat them well and season with salt and pepper. Roast them for 10 mins and then add the garlic cloves to the roasting tray, whole and unpeeled.

Next, prepare the lemon. Peel the rind off, avoiding the bitter white pith underneath, and then finely slice the lemon rind into thin strips. Juice the lemon, put the juice in a bowl along with ½ tsp salt, and then add the lemon rind to this mixture and set aside.

Meanwhile, chop the vegetables. Coat a large skillet/frying pan with olive oil and heat to sauté temperature. Sauté the onions first until soft and translucent, then add the carrots, followed by the squash and zucchini.

Next, add the spices -- ensure the vegetables are well coated in them. Add the tomatoes, aminos and honey, along with the chopped dates and Peppadews or chili. Bring to boiling point and then reduce heat to a simmer. Add the lemon mixture at this point. Simmer for around 15-20 mins.

The sweet potatoes and roasted garlic should now be ready to take out of the oven. Remove the inside of the garlic cloves, but be careful as they will be hot from the oven. Mash the garlic with a little olive oil and then add to the tagine. Add the chickpeas and stir to combine.

Finally, add the sweet potatoes and stir well. Remove from the heat, add the nutritional yeast and salt and pepper to taste.

Serve hot with brown rice, couscous or flatbread. This dish is also great for batch cooking, as it freezes well.

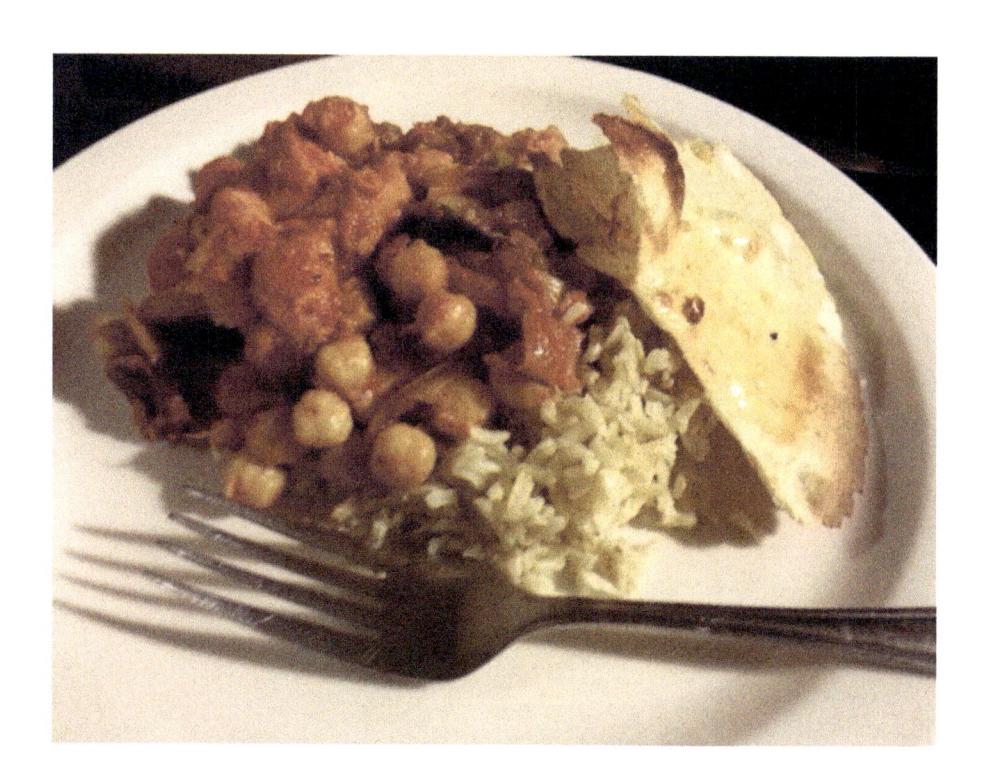

Macaroni no-cheese

This family favorite dish gets a whole food plant-based makeover with this 'cheese' sauce, which is made from cauliflower and silken tofu. The cauliflower gives it the texture, while the tofu adds creaminess. The secret ingredient for the cheesy flavor is nutritional yeast, which is handy because it also gives you all those good B vitamins.

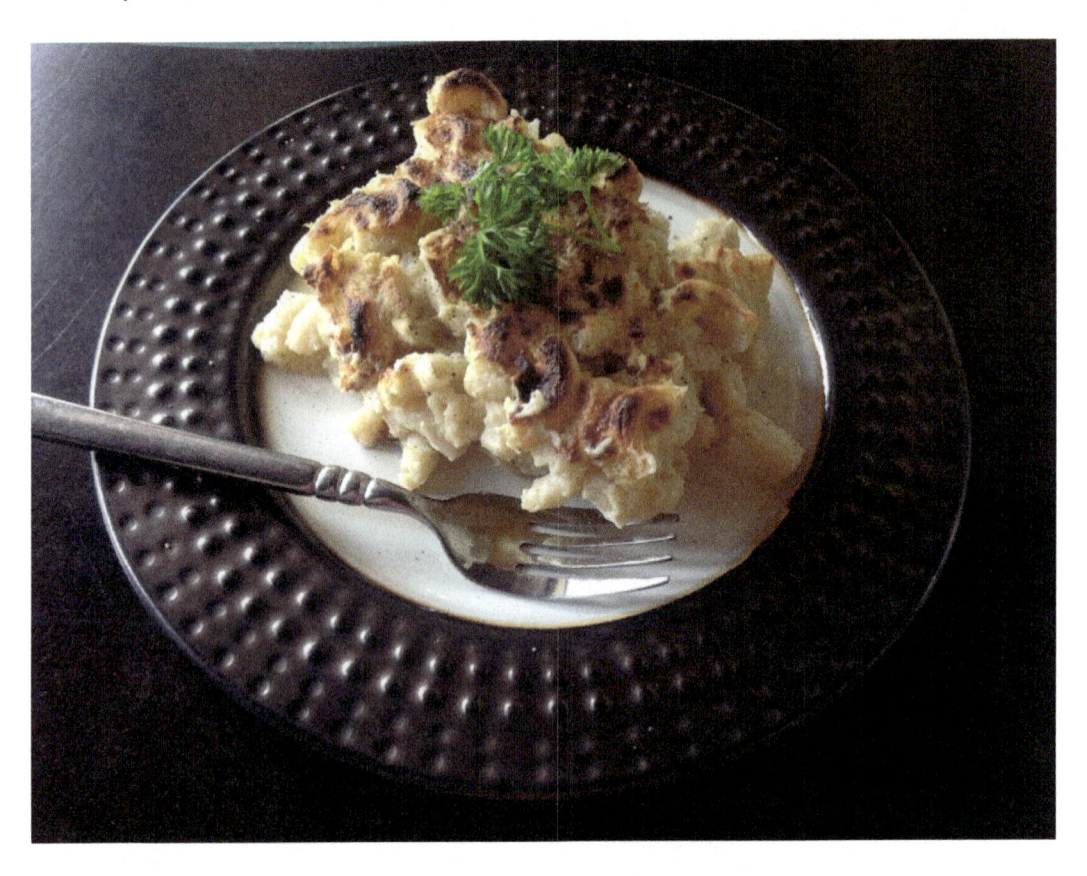

Ingredients
Serves 4-6

½ head of cauliflower, finely chopped
3 cups whole-wheat (or brown rice/quinoa if gluten free) macaroni pasta
1 cup silken tofu, drained
½ cup nutritional yeast
1 tbsp. liquid aminos
1 tsp onion powder or asafetida
1 tsp garlic or celery salt
Juice of ½ lemon
Salt and pepper to taste

Make it

First, cook the cauliflower in salted boiling water or steam it for 10 mins. It should be tender, but not mushy.

Cook the pasta in salted water according to the directions on the pack. With gluten free pasta, it's often helpful to use a little olive oil in the water so it doesn't stick.

Put the cauliflower, tofu, nutritional yeast, aminos, lemon juice and spices into a blender and blitz until creamy.

Preheat the broiler (grill) to its highest setting.

Drain the pasta and then put it back in the pan once it's dry. Add the sauce and heat gently for a couple of minutes, then put the mixture into an ovenproof dish. Once the broiler/grill is heated, put the dish under the heat until browned on top.

Serve hot with a green salad and a sprinkle of chili flakes if you like a little heat with your cheesiness.

Plant-based pizzas

Pizza is one of the foods that UnSupersize Me program participants tell us they miss the most, so here is a healthy, plant-based version of one of the world's favorite fast foods. There are two kinds of pizza here – a more traditional tomato-based veggie pizza and a garlic mushroom version. The cheese is replaced by avocado, which is full of good fats, and a sprinkling of nutritional yeast, which has a slightly cheesy, savory flavor. Why not make both and see which is your favorite?

Traditional veggie

Ingredients
Each pizza serves 8

1 wholegrain pizza crust (must be made with wholegrain flour – if gluten free, look for Mama Mary's, which is made from millet and flax)
Pizza sauce or tomato paste if you can't find a pizza sauce without added sugar.
¼ sweet onion
¼ cup diced red or yellow pepper
¼ cup sliced zucchini
¼ cup sliced yellow squash
¼ cup sliced mushrooms
1 avocado, sliced
Chili flakes/nutritional yeast/salt and pepper to taste

Make it

Preheat the oven according to the instructions on the pizza crust pack.

Spread the pizza crust liberally with the tomato sauce.

Finely chop the veggies and distribute evenly over the crust.

Bake for around 15-20 mins.

Slice the avocado and arrange on top.

Serve with a green salad, season with salt and pepper or chili flakes for a little heat.

Garlic mushroom pizza

This one's for the garlic lovers!

Ingredients
1 wholegrain pizza crust (as for the traditional veggie version)
4 cloves garlic
4 tbsp. olive oil
1 cup chopped mixed mushrooms of your choice – we like a mix of shiitake and button mushrooms, but you can use any you like.
Dried basil and oregano
1 avocado
Salt, pepper and nutritional yeast for topping

Make it

Roast the cloves of garlic in a hot oven for 15 mins until soft and slightly caramelized.

Peel the roasted garlic and mash into a paste. Mix with the olive oil and then spread the mixture over the pizza crust.

Add the mushrooms, herbs and a little salt and pepper.

Bake for 15-20 mins at the required temperature, according to the instructions on the crust.

Arrange the avocado on top.

Sprinkle with salt, pepper and a little nutritional yeast.

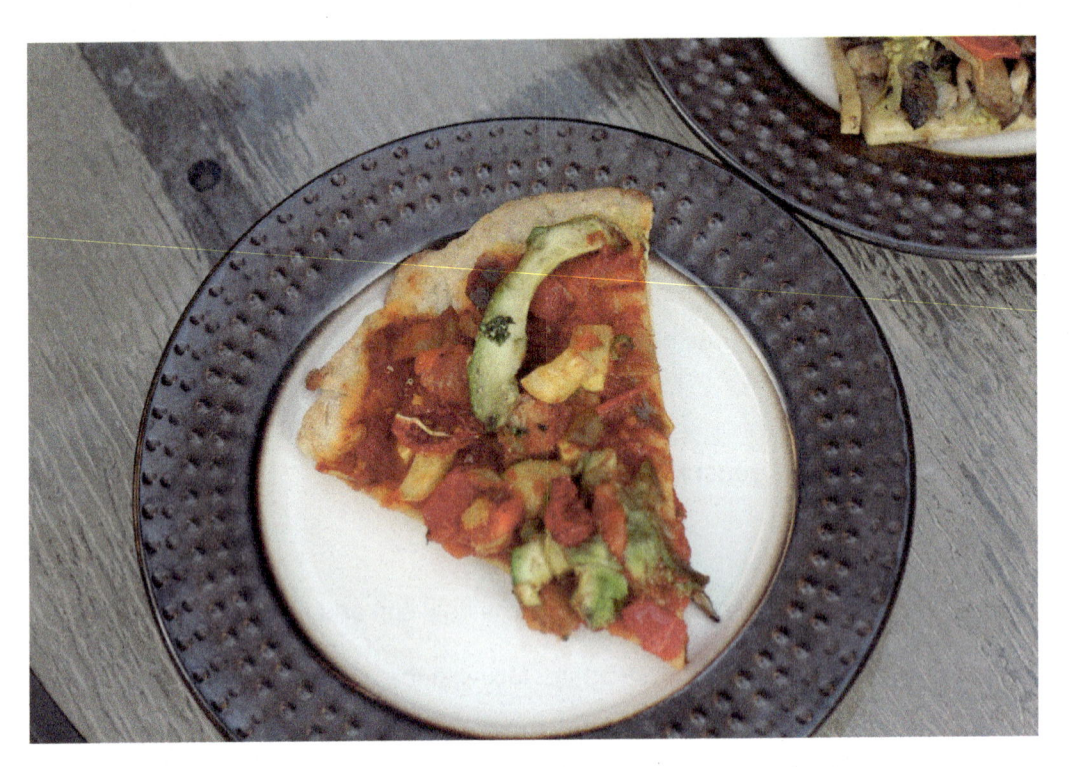

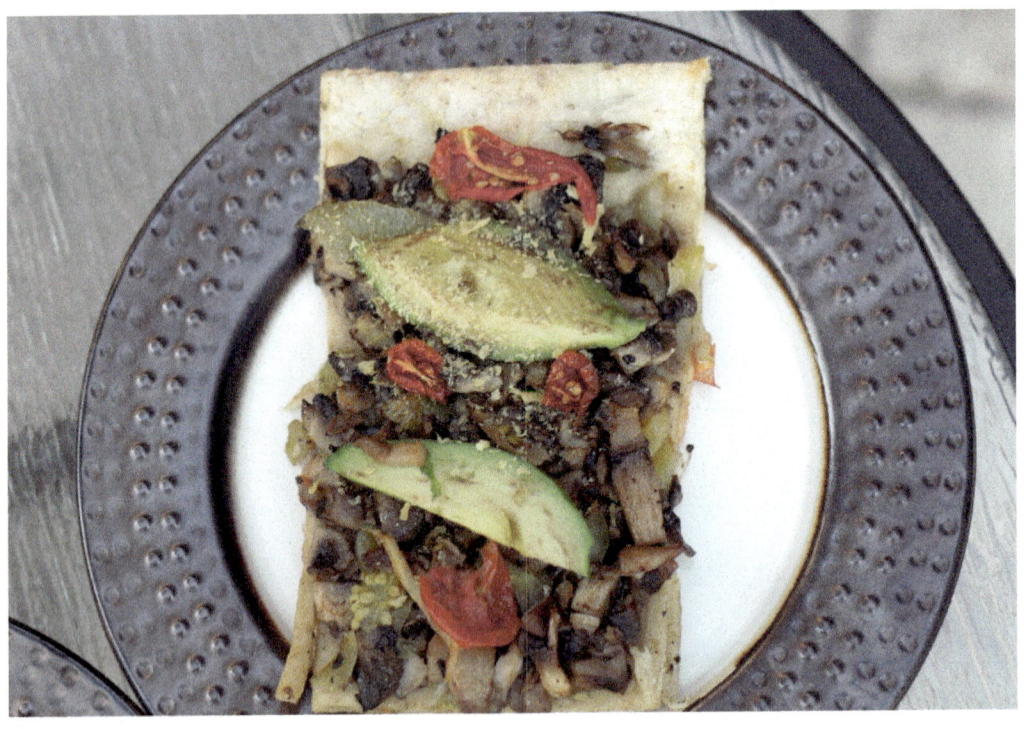

Supercharged salads and sides

Salads are quick, easy and tasty and can be a main event at a meal or a side dish. This selection of salads and sides will ensure that you have plenty of variety with your meals and, of course, get lots of extra veggies in.

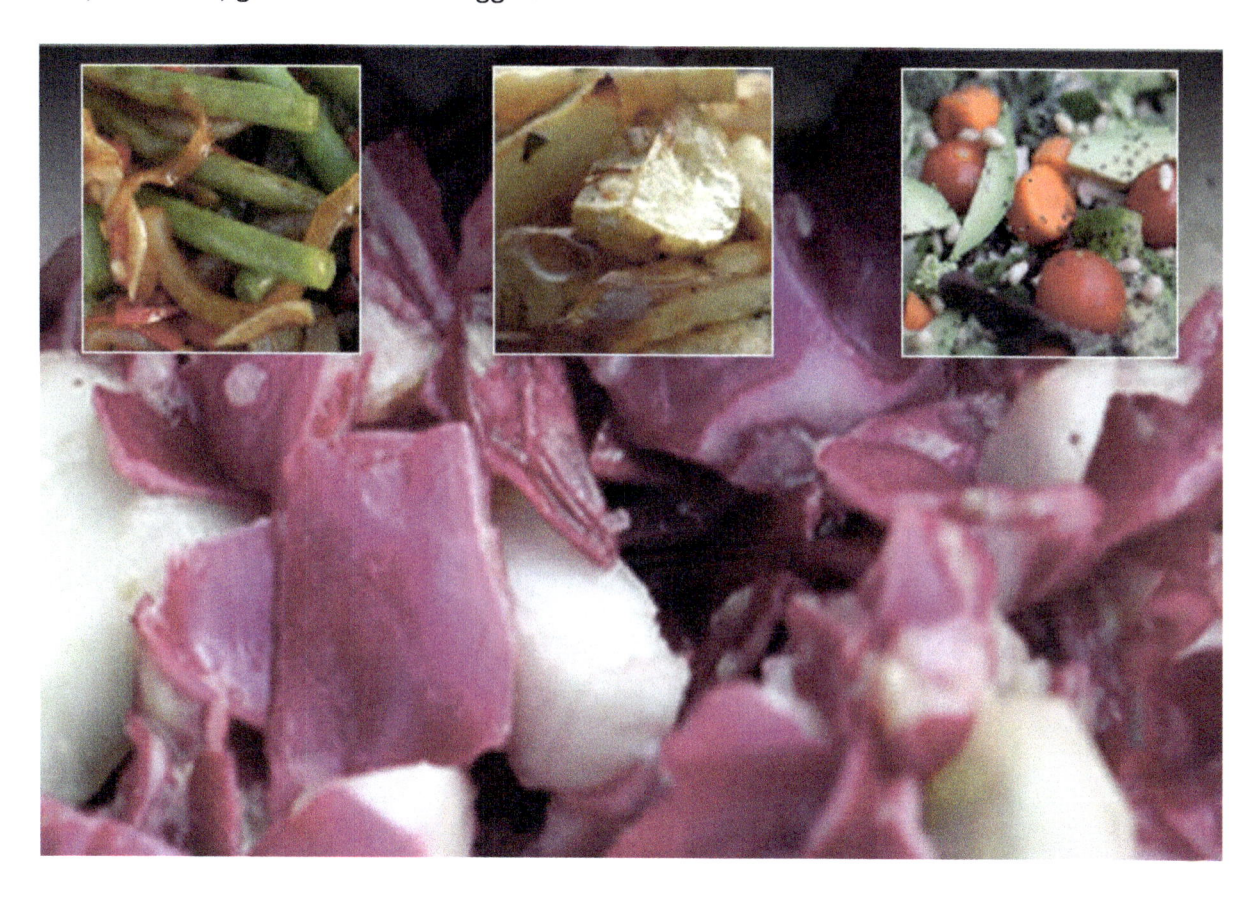

Warm spinach, mushroom and potato salad

Iron Chef Molly Sexton strikes again with this simple but tasty salad that could be served as a side or a light meal on its own. The portabella mushrooms give it some texture (as well as some protein) so it's a nutritionally balanced dish.

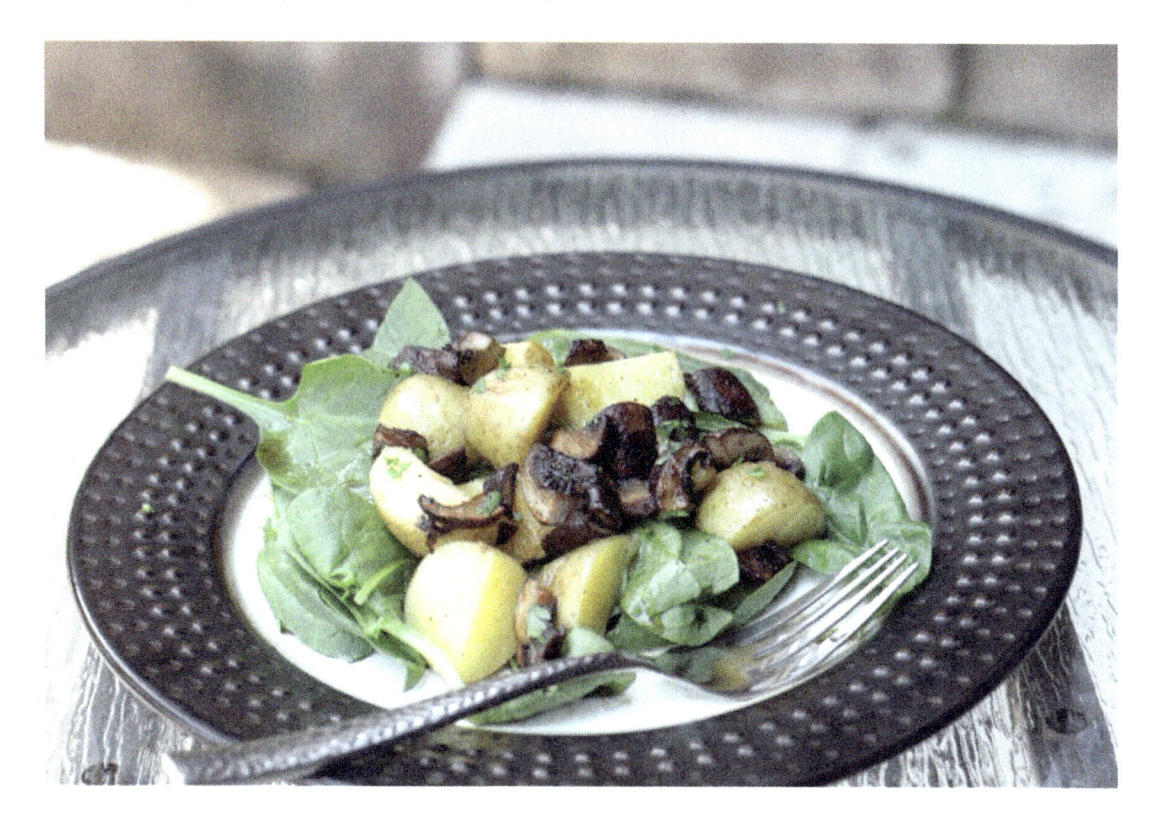

Ingredients
Serves 4

½ kg bag small potatoes (Honey Gold are good, or Jersey Royals if you're on the British side of the pond), diced
1 cup baby portabella mushrooms, diced –
2 tbsp. olive oil
2 cloves garlic, minced
4 cups baby spinach
Salt and pepper to taste

UnSupersize Us signature dressing, to serve

Make it

Preheat oven to 400F/200C/Gas Mark 4

Wash and dice the potatoes and mushrooms.

Peel and mince the cloves of garlic.

On a baking sheet, combine the potatoes, mushrooms, garlic, and olive oil. Add salt and pepper.

Bake for 25-30 minutes at 400, or until the potatoes are soft.

Put 1 cup of the spinach in each of the four salad bowls.

Top with potato and mushroom mixture while still warm.

Add dressing, toss and serve

Carly says...
Don't be afraid of potatoes! Many conventional diets suggest that potatoes are not good for weight loss, but we love them. They provide easily digestible carbohydrate for energy, which is important when you're working out a lot. Potatoes also contain vitamin C and fiber, particularly in the skins.

Pink slaw with avocado

This vibrant and colorful raw salad is a perfect accompaniment to pasta dishes or Mexican meals. The acidity of lime in the dressing adds freshness to any plate and the avocado adds some richness as well as those good fats and Vitamin E, which is good for your skin, hair and nails.

Ingredients
Serves 4
½ of a red cabbage, finely chopped
½ a red onion, finely chopped
1 small cucumber, diced
1 Hass avocado, cut into cubes
¼ cup finely chopped fresh cilantro (coriander)
4 tbsp. white vinegar
1 tbsp. olive oil
Juice of 1 lime
1 tsp liquid aminos
½ tsp agave
Salt and pepper to taste

Make it
Mix all the vegetables together in a large salad bowl.

Add the dressing and combine well.

Leave to rest for 10 min before serving so the flavors blend together.

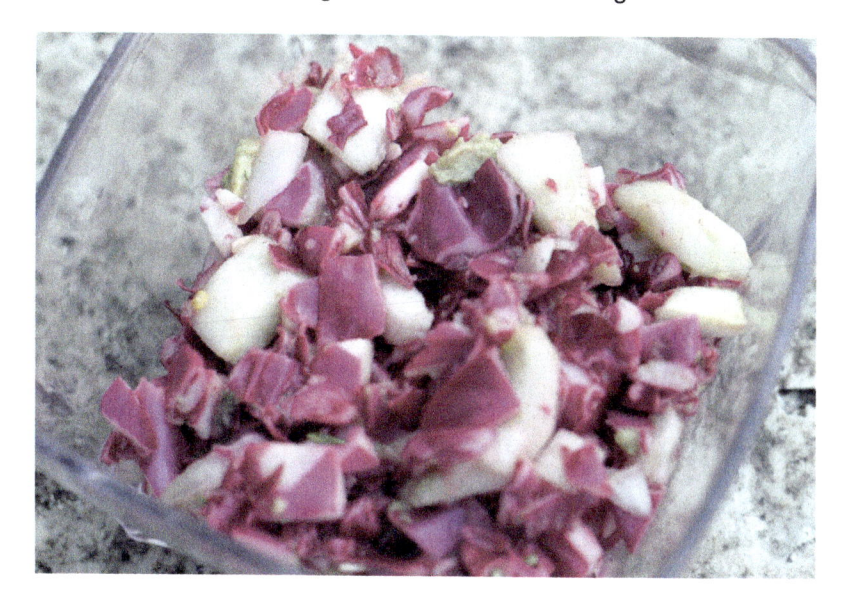

Mushroom, lemon and coriander rice

This dish is ideal for serving with the 'Anything Goes' curry or the sweet potato tagine, since the flavors of coriander and lemon are very versatile. Adding veggies and different flavors to your rice dishes adds variety and texture, ensuring you don't get bored with your plant-based eating. In this dish, the rice is also cooked in vegetable broth (stock) which adds more depth of flavor.

Brown basmati rice is the best kind of brown rice, since it has the lowest glycemic index (GI). This mean it's broken down more slowly, avoiding blood sugar spikes and keeping you fuller for longer.

Ingredients
Serves 4

- 2 cups brown basmati rice
- 4 ½ cups vegetable broth (stock)
- 1 cup diced shallots (or onion if you can't get shallots)
- 2 cups diced mushrooms
- 1 clove garlic, minced
- 2 tsp olive oil
- Rind and juice of 1 lemon
- 2 tbsp. nutritional yeast
- 2 tsp crushed coriander seeds (or powder if you can't get the whole seeds)
- 1 cup chopped fresh coriander leaves
- Salt and pepper to taste

Make it

First, bring the vegetable broth to the boil on the stovetop for the rice (unless you're using a rice cooker, in which case simply add the ingredients and set the timer). Add the rice and simmer for around 25 mins.

Meanwhile, dice the shallots and mushrooms and mince the garlic. Sauté the shallots in the olive oil first, until they start to soften and become translucent. Add the mushrooms, garlic and crushed coriander seeds and stir to combine. Sauté for another 3-5 mins and set aside.

Finely grate the lemon rind, then squeeze the juice out. Roughly chop the fresh coriander.

When the rice is cooked, drain it well. Return the shallots and mushrooms to the heat and add the rice in slowly, stirring as you go. Add the lemon rind, juice, and nutritional yeast, and add salt and pepper to taste.

Finally, remove from the heat and stir the fresh coriander through.

Chili garlic green beans

The plain old green bean is given a makeover in this slightly sweet and spicy Asian-style stir-fried dish. You can vary the heat to suit your tastes by using different kinds of chili pepper, according to how hot you like it. If you're a heat lover (like Carly and Liz) go for bird's eye chilies, but if you like something milder, go for Poblano or Serrano peppers.

Ingredients
Serves 2

- 1 small onion, sliced finely
- 2 cups green beans, with the tips removed
- 1-2 fresh chili peppers (de-seed them if you want it milder)
- 2 cloves garlic, finely sliced
- 1 tsp coconut oil
- 2 tbsp. soy sauce (use tamari if gluten free is required)
- 2 tbsp. rice or sherry vinegar
- 1 tbsp. agave

Make it

Heat the coconut oil in a wok (a frying pan/skillet will do if you don't have one) on a high heat until you see the oil start to ripple slightly (but don't let it start to smoke!)

Add the onions and stir fry for 1-2 mins, keeping them moving.

Add the green beans and stir fry for another minute. Add the chili and garlic and stir fry for around 30 secs. With stir frying, the trick is to keep the heat high and keep everything moving in the pan so nothing burns.

Add the wet ingredients and stir to combine. Stir fry for another minute or two and let the liquid reduce a little.

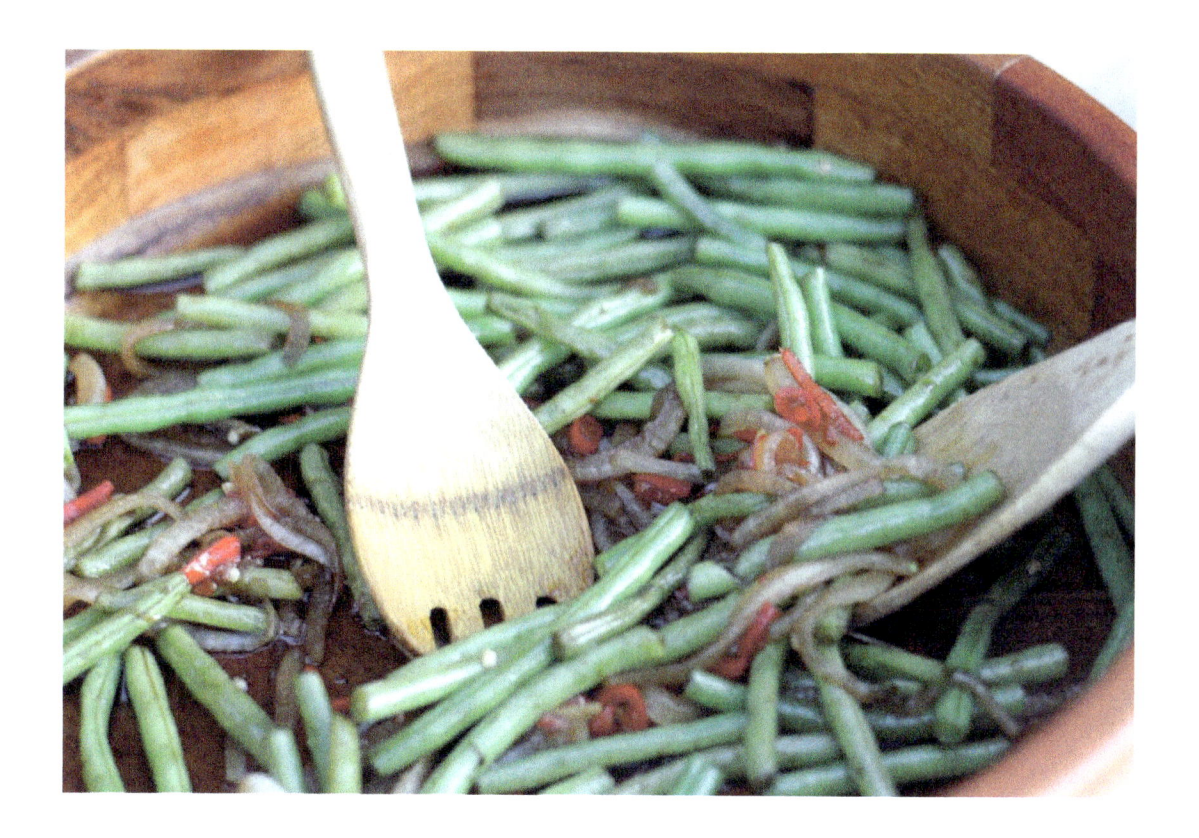

A note about chili
In some studies, Chili has been found to boost metabolism (that is, the rate at which the body burns calories from food) after eating. It's all down to the chemical capsaicin, which is what gives chili peppers their heat. It's not a substitute for hard work in the gym though, so don't get any ideas!

Yucca fries

Yucca (also called cassava) is a Caribbean, Central American and African staple food. It's a starchy, fibrous root that's white in color. Cassava has more Vitamin C and fiber than potatoes. That includes a fiber called inulin, which is good for feeding the beneficial bacteria in your gut and contributing to good digestive balance, so it's an excellent choice. Cooking it from fresh takes a lot of preparation, however, so we prefer to use frozen cassava as it's easier to work with and takes less time to cook.

Ingredients
Serves 4-6

1kg bag frozen yucca (also called cassava)
2-3 tbsp. good quality olive oil
Sea salt
Nutritional yeast/chili flakes for serving (optional)

Make it

Boil the chunks of yucca for around 30 mins until soft. Drain well and leave to dry on kitchen roll for 10-15 mins

Heat the oil on a flat baking tray in a preheated oven (200C/375F or Gas 6)

When it's sufficiently cooled and dried, chop it up into chunky chip-sized pieces. As you chop it, remove any of the thick fibrous strands that come from the middle of the root. These are not too palatable and will make your fries chewy.

Add the yucca to the preheated oil. It may sizzle a bit. Toss the yucca in the oil so it's well coated and sprinkle with salt.

Return it to the oven and bake for approx. 20 mins, turning halfway through to ensure even cooking.

Sprinkle with salt and nutritional yeast before serving - or add some chili flakes if you like some heat!

Citrus salsa Fresca

This salsa is a lovely summer dish – the fresh and zingy flavors of lime and cilantro make it a great accompaniment to Mexican dishes and it's full of healthy raw veggies too.

Ingredients:
Serves 4

5-6 medium to large tomatoes chopped
½ head of red cabbage chopped
½ sweet yellow onion chopped
½ bunch fresh cilantro chopped
4-5 limes freshly squeezed
1-3 of your choice of fresh hot peppers (for example jalapeños or serrano if you prefer a milder pepper, or habanero, tabasco, or cayenne if you like it hotter), deseeded and chopped small. If you don't like any heat, try using baby bell or Anaheim peppers -- they have the sweetness without the spice.
Salt to taste.

Make it
Chop all the ingredients finely and combine in a large bowl.

Squeeze the lime juice over.

Stir well and season with salt to taste.

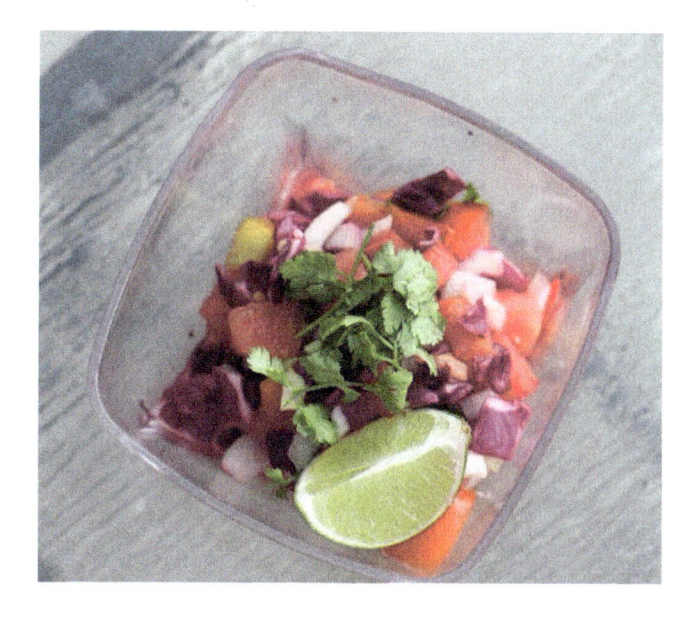

Perfect-every-time potato fries

Think you can't eat fries on a whole food plant-based diet? These crunchy, moreish potato fries will make you think again. They're cooked in the oven rather than deep-fried, so they're much healthier, but they still have the crispy outside and soft fluffy inside that we all love.

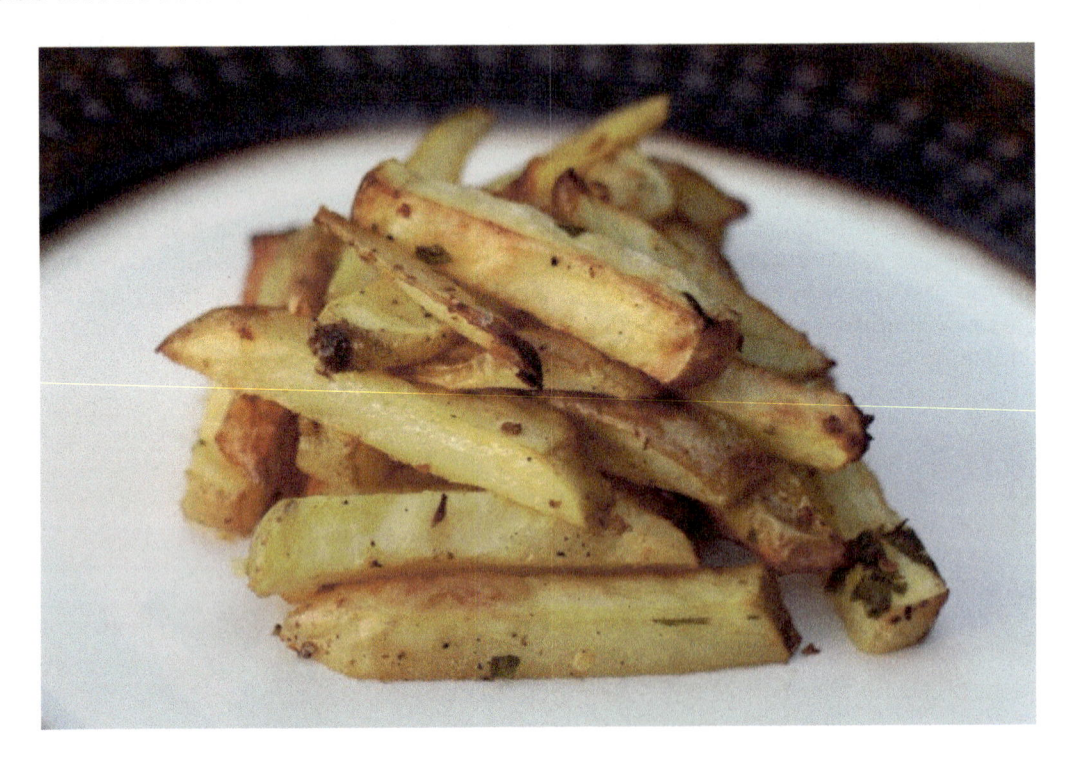

Ingredients
Serves 4

6-8 medium sized white potatoes, skin on
olive oil
Salt

Make it

Preheat the oven to 375F/220C/Gas 6.

Cut the potatoes into fry-sized chunks. You can choose how chunky you want them to be, but keep in mind that larger fries will take longer to cook.

Coat the bottom of a baking tray with olive oil. Heat in the oven for 2-3 mins.

Add the fries to the pan and shake well to coat the potatoes

Bake for 20-25 mins, turning once to ensure even cooking.

Serve as a side with any of our delicious main dishes.

Fire roasted tomatoes

This is an amazingly simple side dish that showcases the lovely sweet taste of fresh ripe tomatoes. Tomatoes are actually healthier for you when cooked, because the cooking process releases a substance called lycopene, which is a beneficial antioxidant.

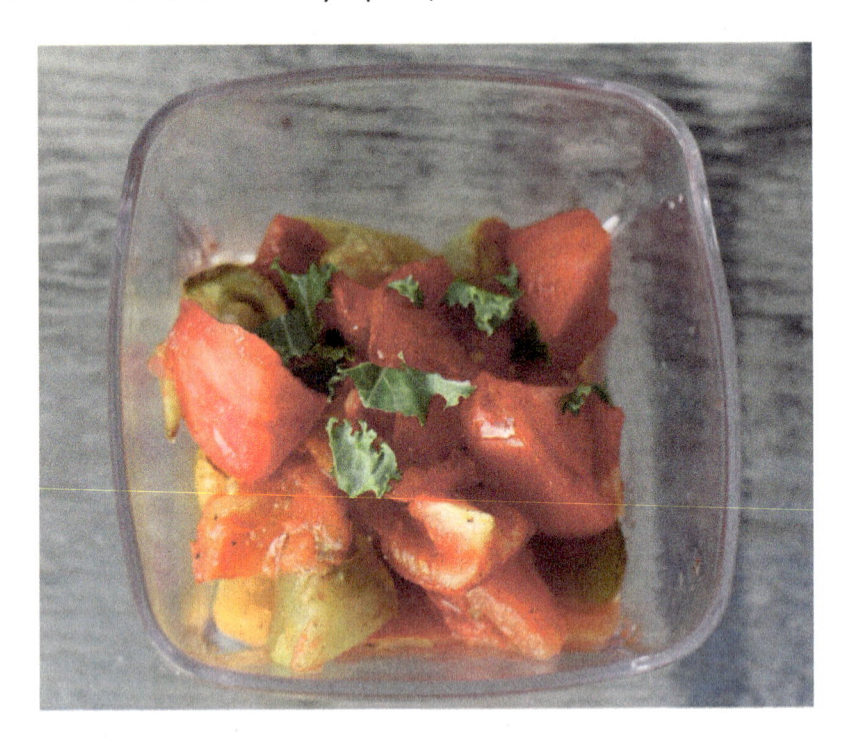

Ingredients
Serves 4

10-12 ripe tomatoes (use more if using a smaller variety)
1 tbsp. olive oil
Salt

Make it

Preheat the oven to 300F/175C/Gas Mark 4

Chop the tomatoes into quarters

Place in a mixing bowl. Add olive oil and a sprinkle of salt. Mix to ensure the tomatoes are evenly coated.

Roast for 20 mins on a baking sheet, turning half way through

Dips and dressings to die for

Dressing maketh the salad, as we say around here. It's important to get your veggies in, so it's essential that they taste great. The right dressing or a healthy dip can do wonders for a raw salad or a plate of raw veggies, so here's a few that you'll find yourself making time and time again.

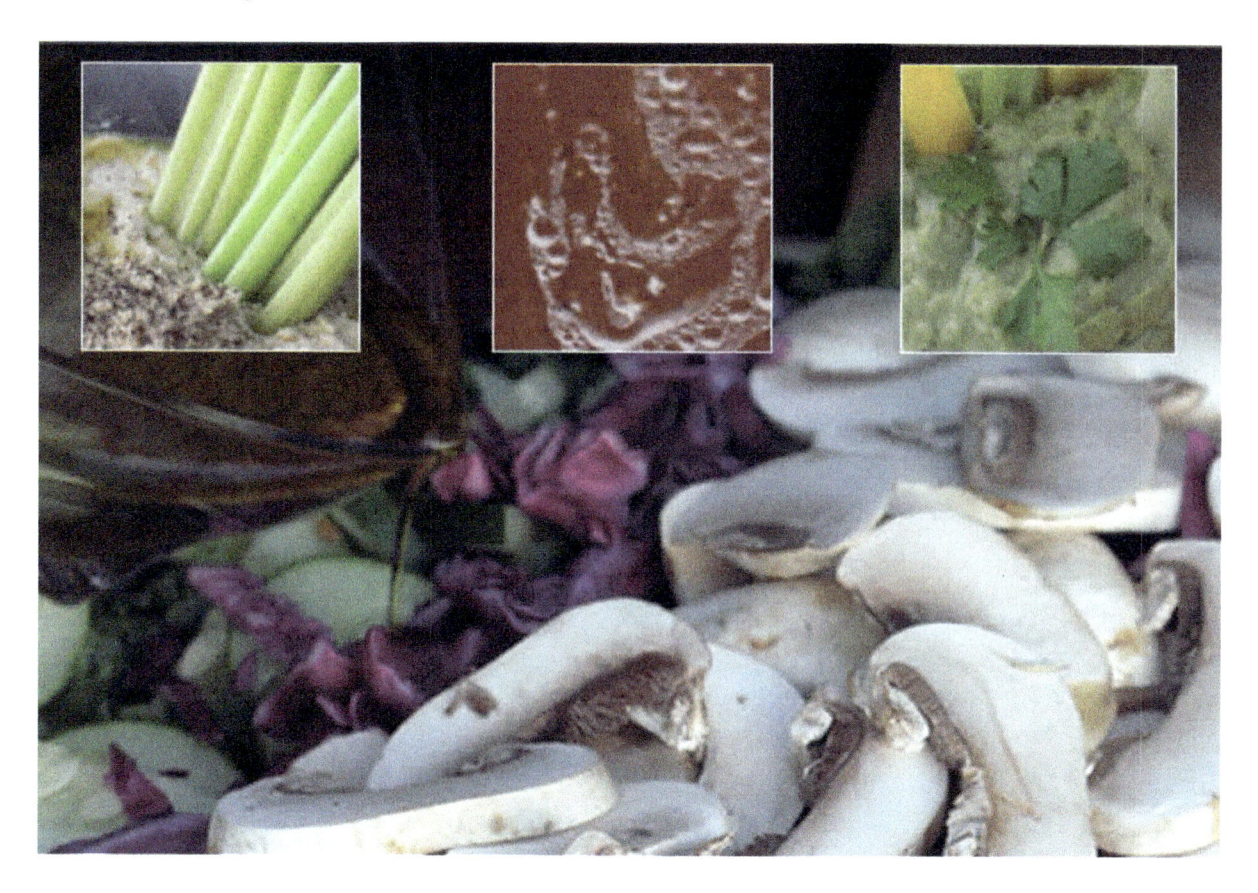

Hummus

It wouldn't be a plant-based cookbook without hummus – this Middle Eastern dip/spread based on chickpeas is one of those rare foods that everyone seems to agree on, no matter what their dietary preferences. Even die-hard Paleo aficionados have been known to bend the rules on legumes to accommodate hummus, it's *that* good.

Of course, you can buy hummus in stores. The problem with those is that they usually contain nasties like preservatives, vegetable oils and even added sugar. Unless you're in the UK and live close to a Marks and Spencer, that is, where they do a hummus made with extra-virgin olive oil. This is the only store-bought hummus we've found so far that hits all the whole food plant-based buttons, but we think it's much easier and cheaper to make your own.

Ingredients
Serves 4 (okay, we'll admit it, it probably only serves 2 around here because we're hummus addicts, so double the quantities if you want it to last more than five minutes)

- 1 can chickpeas (garbanzos), drained (save the liquid)
- 2 tbsp. extra virgin olive oil
- 1 clove garlic, minced
- Juice of 1 lemon
- 2 tbsp. tahini (check the ingredients for added oil, there should be no ingredients other than sesame seeds)
- 2 tbsp. nutritional yeast
- 1 tsp sea salt

Make it
How easy is this – just drop all those ingredients into a blender and whizz up until it's a smooth paste. If it seems a little too thick and the blender struggles to process it, you can add a little of the water from the can of chickpeas.

Serve with raw vegetables for dipping, spread on sprouted grain toast, use as a filling for baked potatoes…once you've made your own, we don't think you'll ever go back to store bought.

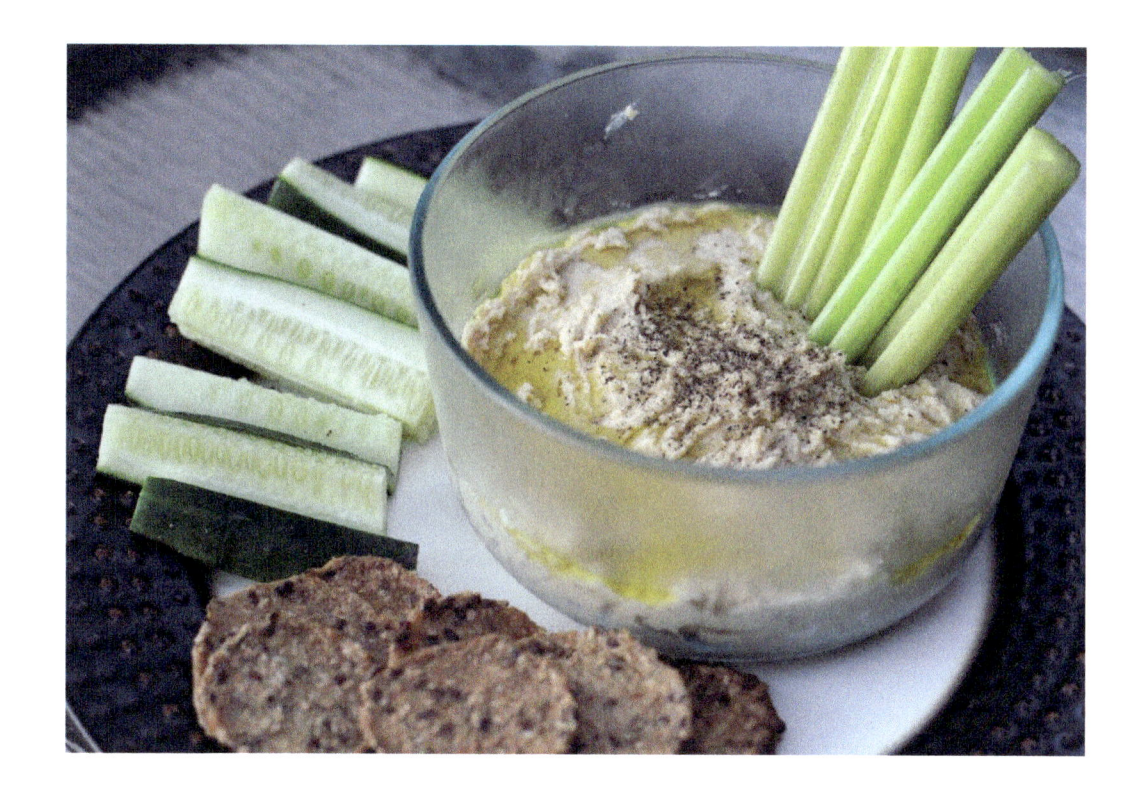

Variations

Once you're confident with the basic recipe, you can try switching it up and adding different flavors. You could also make hummus with cannellini or butter beans instead of chickpeas.

The Mediterranean – add 2 tsp sundried tomato paste to the mix and garnish with sliced olives

The Moroccan – garnish with dukkah spice and chopped preserved lemons

The Italian – Add fresh basil leaves to the mix, sprinkle with pine nuts and a drizzle of olive oil

Old Smokey – add smoked paprika and a little tomato paste

The Mexican – Add chopped jalapeno peppers into your mixture. If you like it even hotter, sprinkle chili flakes on top.

Holy guacamole

Guacamole is a traditional Mexican dish made from avocado, flavored with garlic, lime and a subtle hit of chili. It's a great accompaniment to Molly Sexton's No'Chos on page XX, or served with raw vegetables as a light lunch, starter or side dish.

Ingredients
Serves 4

3 ripe avocadoes
½ small onion, diced small
1 medium tomato, diced small
1 clove garlic, crushed
1 fresh chili pepper, diced small – habanero if you like it hot, jalapeño or serrano if you like it milder – or if you don't like heat at all, leave the chili out altogether
Juice of 3 limes
½ tsp sea salt

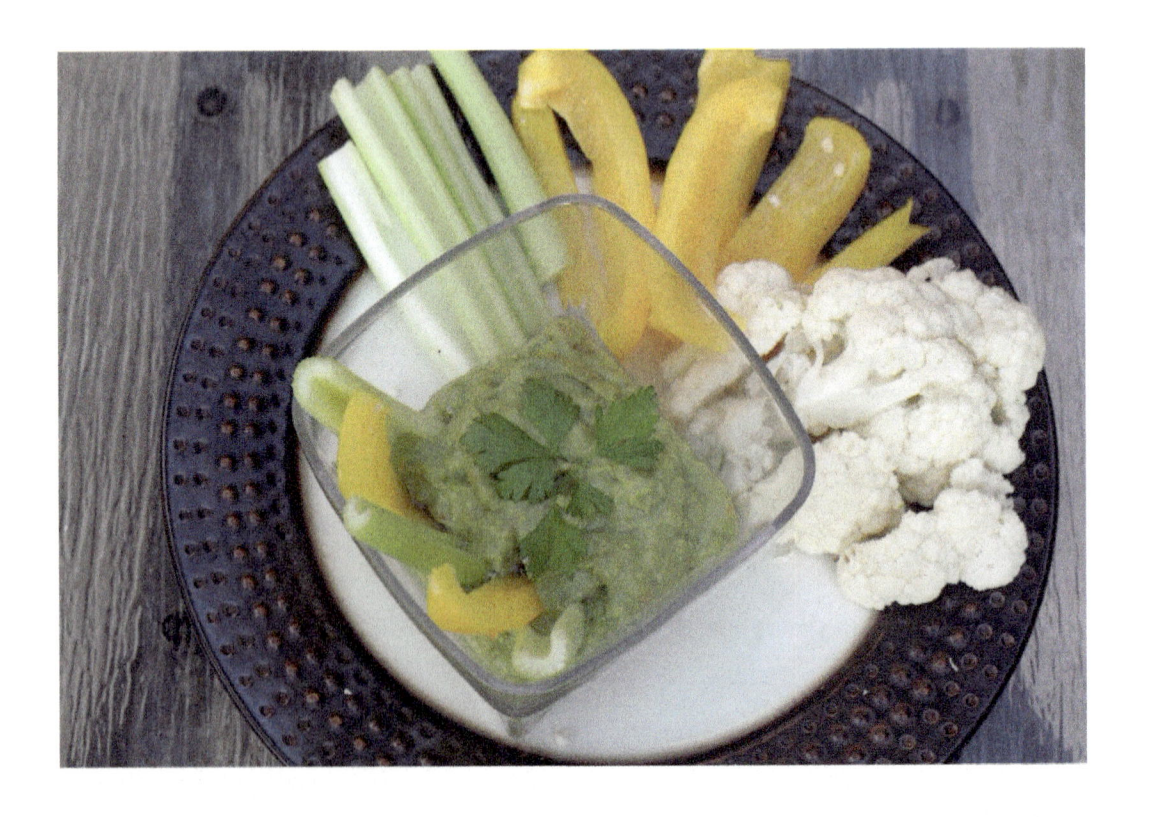

Make it

Peel and mash the avocadoes in a bowl. You can mash them to a puree consistency or leave it slightly chunky, depending how you like the texture

Finely dice the onion and tomato and stir through the mashed avocado, followed by the garlic and chili

Juice the limes and add the lime juice gradually. We like our guac with a good kick of lime, but if you prefer it creamier, you can use a little less of the lime juice.

Add salt to taste.

Lemon tahini dressing

Molly Patrick is a whole food plant-based nutritional guru who knows everything about how to make plants taste awesome. This lemon-tahini dressing is one of her most popular recipes – it's so good that it's known as "tahini crack" among the members in the Clean Food Dirty Girl Facebook group. This is quite sweet, so if you prefer your dressings with more acidity, use fewer dates and a little more lemon juice. Thanks, Molly!

Ingredients
Serves 4

½ cup tahini
Juice of 1 lemon
2 garlic cloves, chopped
6 dates, pitted and simmered in water for 10 mins (if the dates are huge or you like it less sweet, use 4 dates)
¾ tsp sea salt
¾ cup water

Make it

Drain the water from the boiled dates.

Place all of the ingredients in your blender and blend until creamy and smooth, about one full minute.

Use this as salad dressing, pour it over roast veggies, use it as mayo and to drizzle over tacos and burritos. You can use this sauce for any damn thing and it will be delicious.

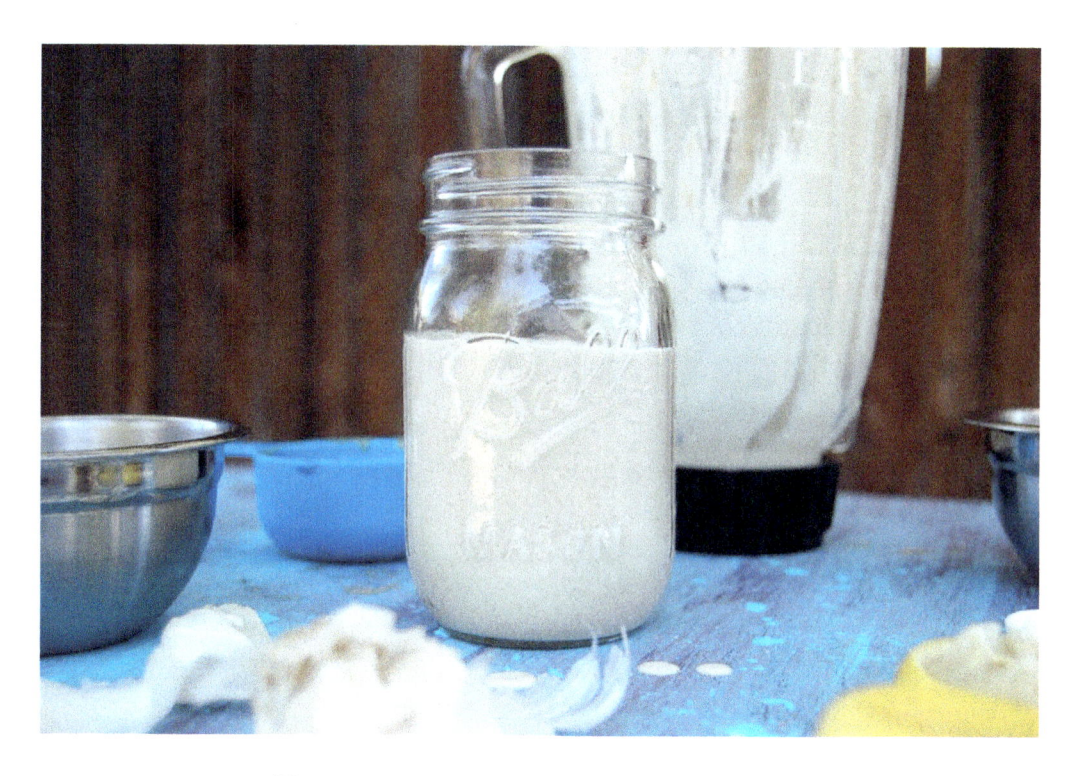

Photo by Molly Patrick, used with permission

UnSupersize Us signature dressing

This dressing was a hit with everyone in the *UnSupersize Us* movie, so it became affectionately known as the *UnSupersize Us* dressing since it was requested at pretty much every meal we all had together. This is a perfect example of the gourmet chef's golden rules – a combination of sweet, salty and sour flavors to appeal to the palate and bring those green salads to life.

Ingredients
Enough for a large green salad to serve 4 people – will also keep in the fridge for a couple of days.

2 tbsp. liquid aminos
2 tbsp. balsamic vinegar
1 tbsp. olive oil
1 tbsp. agave
Pinch of salt and black pepper

Make it

Combine ingredients and stir well, ensuring the agave is dissolved fully. Pour over a fresh raw salad with plenty of greens and enjoy.

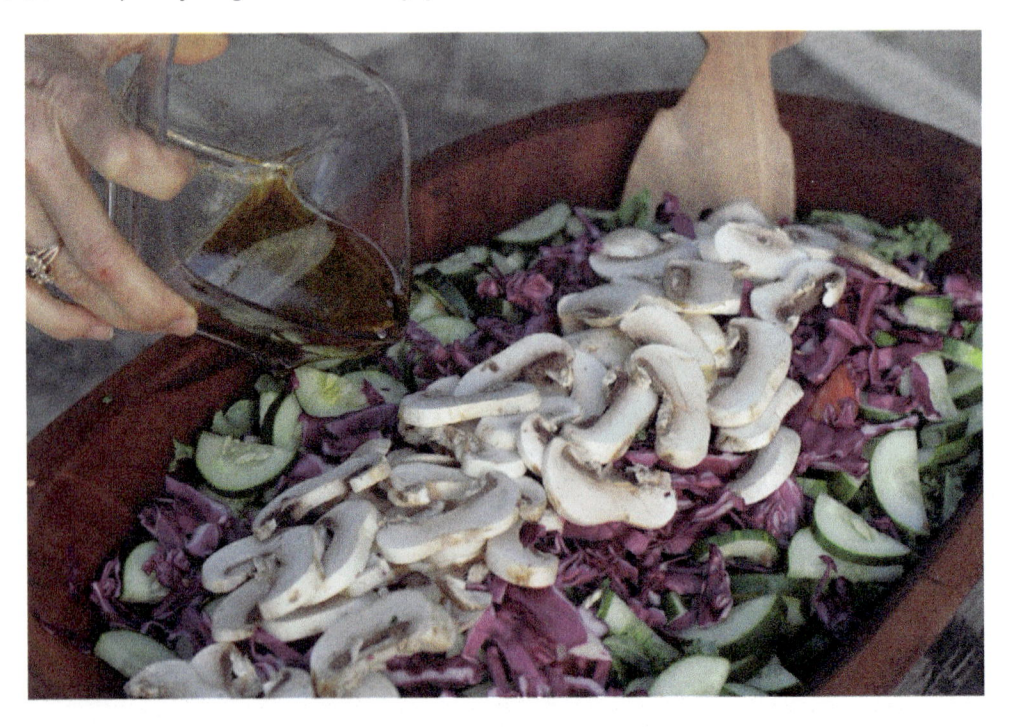

Balsamic vinaigrette

We're all about making salads interesting by packing plenty of flavor into our dressings. This is a traditional Italian style dressing that will go well on most salads and is a healthy alternative to ready-made vinaigrette dressings, which often use vegetable oils and are sweetened with refined sugar. This dressing is a great match for a side salad to go with Sandy's sundried tomato pesto pasta.

Ingredients
Makes enough for a large salad to serve 4 people.

2 tbsp. olive oil
2 tbsp. balsamic vinegar
1 tbsp. agave
1 tsp wholegrain mustard
Pinch of salt and pepper

Make it

Combine ingredients and mix well, ideally whisking with a fork so the oil starts to thicken just a little. This gives it a richer, silkier texture that will mimic the kind of vinaigrette dressing you'd find in restaurants.

Pour over salad, toss well to coat all those lovely leaves and raw veggies and enjoy.

Delicious desserts and bakes

Yes, you can have your plant-based cake and eat it with this selection of desserts and baked goodies. Although we don't advocate eating this kind of thing every day, we do recognize that there are special occasions that will come up, or people will come around for dinner and everyone wants to be able to serve something a little bit indulgent. We've tried to come up with some healthier alternatives that are free of animal ingredients and refined sugar.

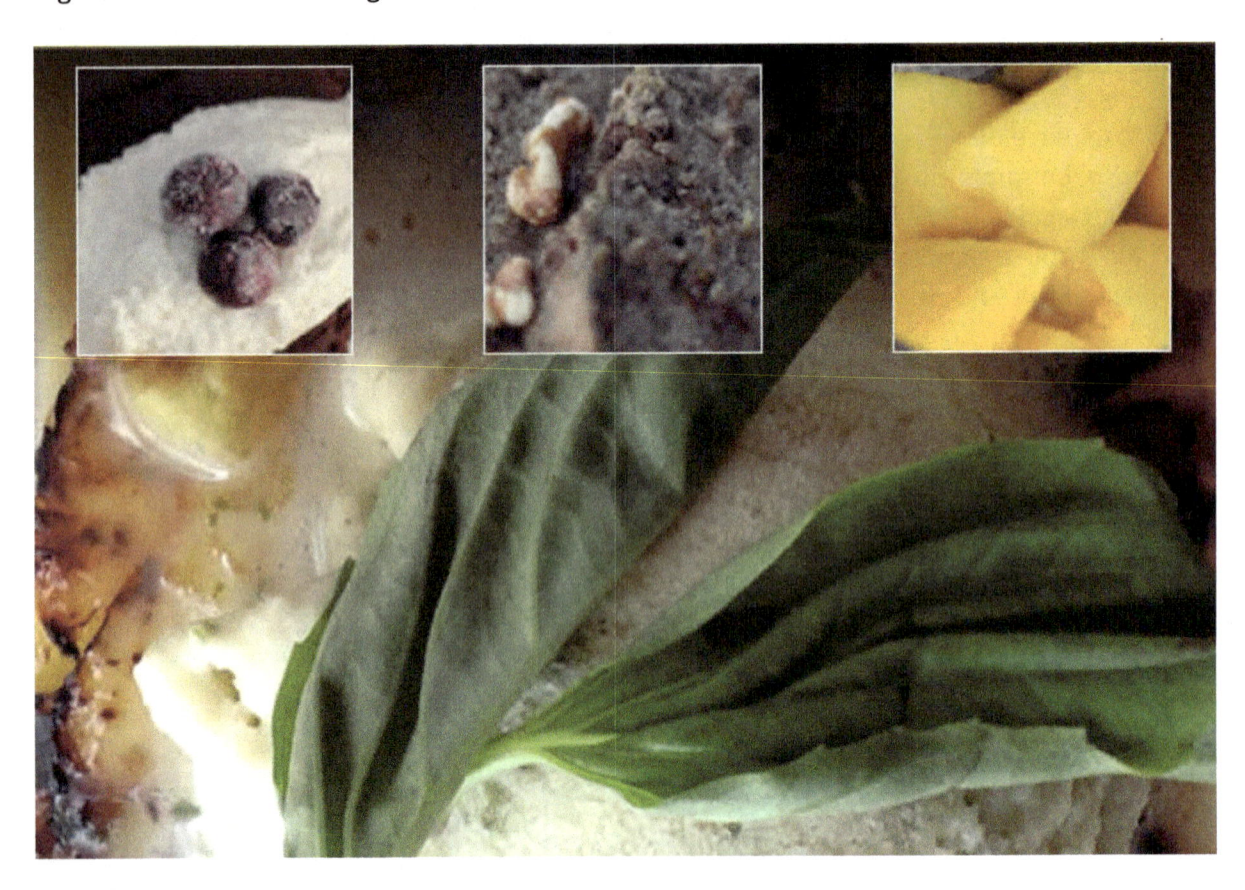

Coconut chia pudding with mango

Chia seeds are a great source of fiber, protein and healthy Omega 3 fats that benefit your skin, joints and brain function. Because of the fiber content in the seeds, when combined with liquid, chia seeds swell and soften and that makes them ideal for making this pudding, which is similar to tapioca pudding often seen in Asian cuisine. This is a light, summery dessert with the flavors of Southeast Asia.

Ingredients
Makes 4 puddings

½ cup chia seeds
1 cup full fat coconut cream (you can skim off the cream from a can of coconut milk for this)
1 cup dairy free unsweetened coconut milk (found in the fridge section of most supermarkets)
¼ cup maple syrup or agave
1 tsp vanilla extract
1 ripe mango, flesh removed and diced
Juice of ½ a lime

Make it

Combine the chia seeds with the coconut cream, maple syrup/agave and vanilla. Stir well and then put in the refrigerator for 4 hours to allow the chia seeds to absorb the liquid.

Remove the flesh from the mango and dice finely. Put in a bowl and then squeeze the lime juice over.

When the pudding is set, spoon into equal portions in individual bowls and then top each one with the mango mixture. Enjoy chilled.

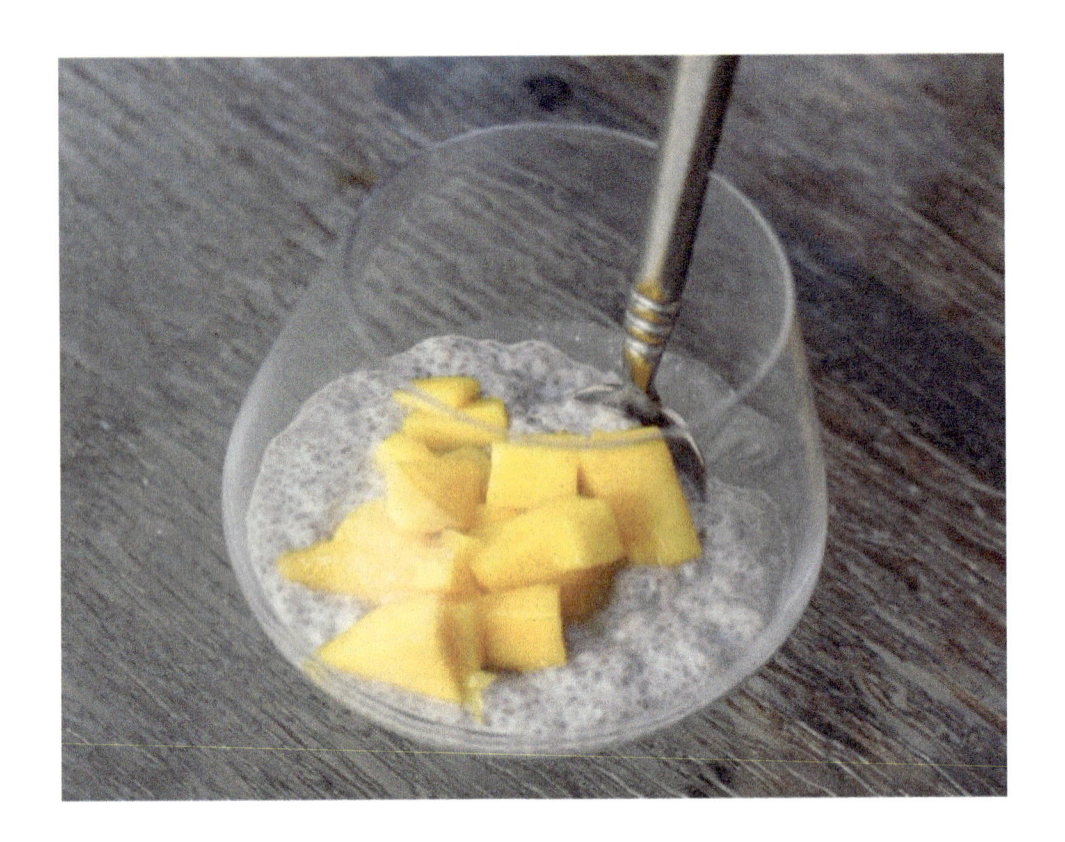

A note about chia seeds
The reason chia is a superfood is because these little seeds are protein packed! They also contain Omega 3 fats, which we need for brain function. Chia seeds also contain fiber, which is good for the digestive system. They are more easily digested when they are either soaked or ground, so try using them for puddings, smoothies, or mixing them into oatmeal.

Thai basil and lemongrass ice cream

We're staying in Southeast Asia for this coconut milk-based ice cream dessert by UK-based food blogger Steve Dent, which is rich and creamy but also fresh and fragrant with traditional Thai herbs that can lend themselves to sweet or savory dishes. This is a perfect dessert to round off a spicy meal and you could accompany it with some grilled pineapple (as shown below) or a fresh tropical fruit salad.

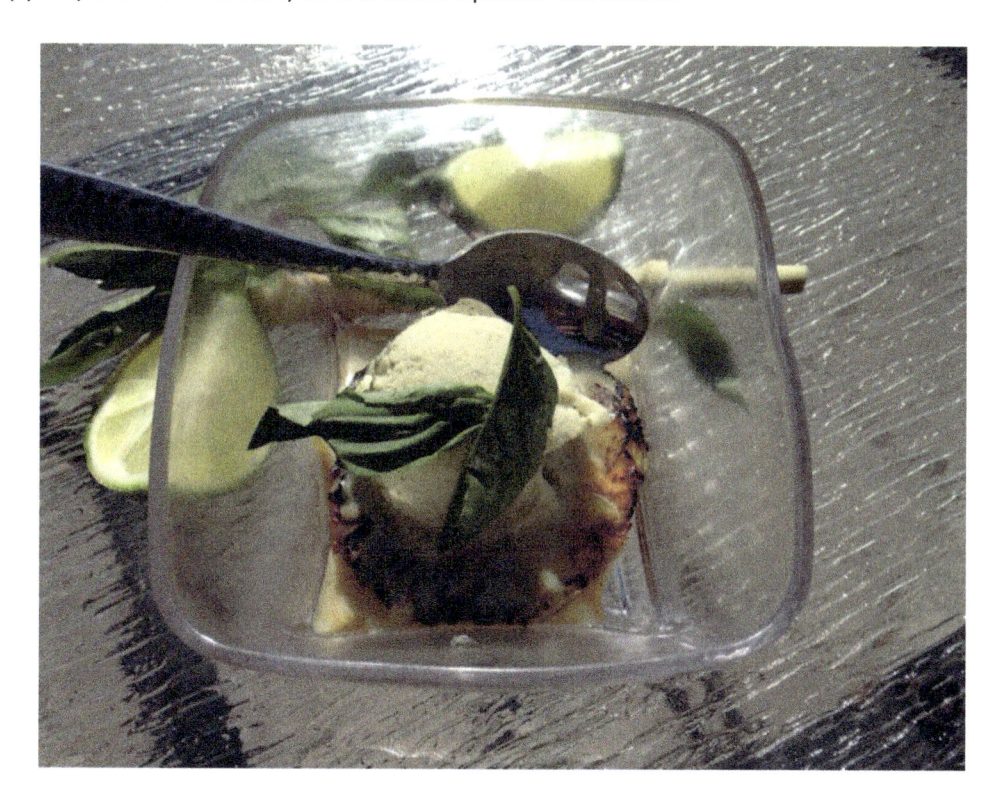

You can buy Thai basil and lemongrass from most Asian supermarkets.

Ingredients

800 ml (2 cans) full fat organic coconut milk
6 fresh lemongrass stalks
10g (about 2 tbsp.) fresh Thai basil leaves
Pinch sea salt
150 ml maple syrup

Make it

Crush the lemongrass stalks with the flat of a large knife, pressing down until you hear a satisfying crack.

Give the cans of coconut milk a good shake to combine the contents, then pour the coconut milk into a pan. Add the maple syrup, sea salt and crushed lemongrass stalks. Place the pan over a low heat and slowly heat up, stirring every so often. When the milk reaches simmering point, remove it from the heat and set it to one side to cool completely.

Bring a pan of water to the boil. Drop the Thai basil leaves into the boiling water, then quickly stir and immediately drain into a sieve before plunging the leaves into ice cold water. Drain again and then gently squeeze the excess moisture from the blanched leaves. Chop the leaves roughly.

When the coconut milk has cooled to room temperature, pour it through a sieve into a blender, discarding the lemongrass stalks. Add the chopped Thai basil leaves to the coconut milk, then process in the blender for 2-3 minutes until fully combined. You should end up with a pale green liquid of uniform consistency.

Pour the ice cream liquid into a large jug and chill in the fridge for an hour.

Pour the chilled ice cream mixture into an ice cream maker and churn. Once it is starting to set, tip the ice cream out into a freezer proof container. Cover the container with a lid and freeze for at least 4 hours. Remove the ice cream from the freezer and leave to stand at room temperature for 15 minutes before serving.

Mayan-spiced chocolate muffins with fudge frosting

Who doesn't love a chocolate muffin? This is a nice easy one bowl recipe, which makes moist, rich muffins and combines the traditional Mayan flavors of chili and chocolate with a fudgy frosting – but most importantly, they're plant-based and refined sugar free. Raw cacao also adds an antioxidant injection to these delicious morsels – it's much higher in beneficial flavones, the chemical compound in the cacao bean that's good for you, than chocolate that's been heat treated.

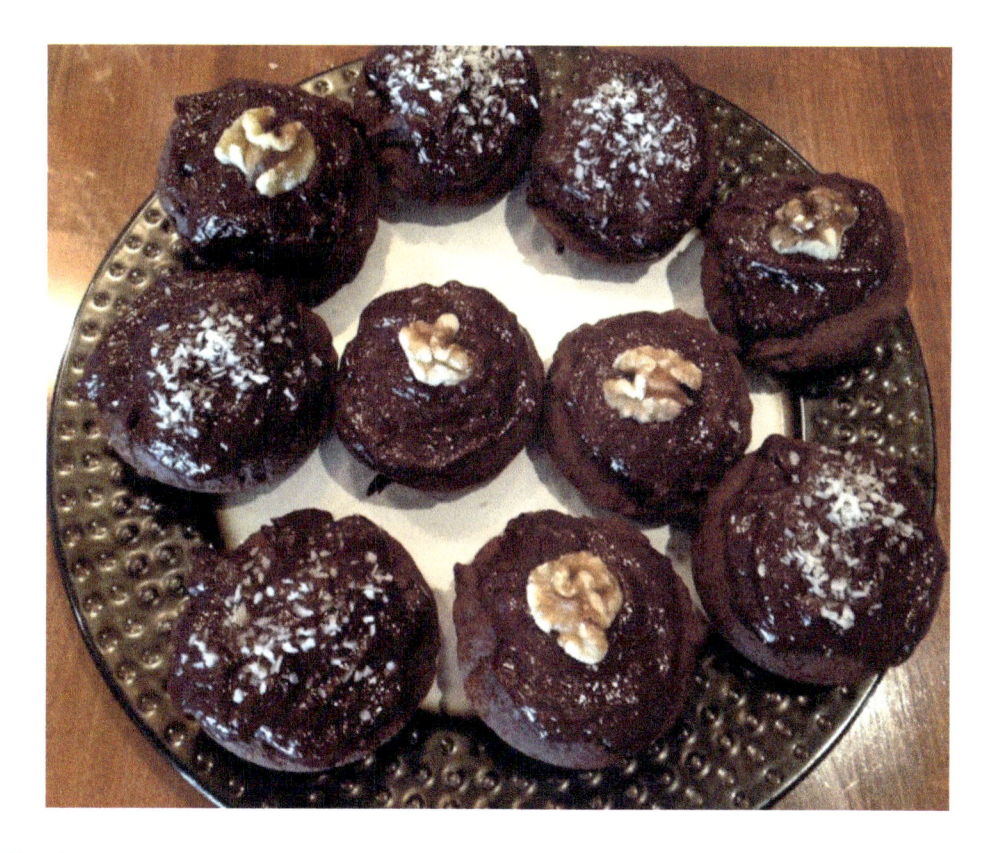

Ingredients
Makes 12 small muffins or 6 large

Muffins
3/4 cup ground almonds
¾ cup brown rice flour
2 tbsp. coconut oil
1/2 cup maple syrup/agave
10 tbsp. raw cacao powder
2 tbsp. dairy free milk
2 flax eggs

1 tsp vanilla extract
1 tsp bicarb soda
½ tsp cayenne pepper
pinch of sea salt

Frosting
5 tbsp. raw cacao powder
2 tbsp. dairy free milk
2 tbsp. maple syrup/agave
2 tbsp. almond butter
pinch of sea salt

Make it

Preheat the oven to 350F/180C and line a 12-cup muffin tin with muffin cases

Make the flax eggs by combining 2 tbsp. flaxseed meal with 6 tbsp. water. Leave to stand for 10-15 min.

Measure and combine the ground almonds, brown rice flour, cacao powder, cayenne, bicarb soda and salt. Mix well – you could use a stand mixer, if you have one.

Add the oil, maple syrup, flax eggs, milk and vanilla and mix well to combine.

Divide the mixture equally between the muffin cases. Bake for 20-25 mins or until a skewer inserted into the middle of one of the muffins comes out clean.

Allow to cool.

Make the frosting by combining the cacao, dairy free milk, syrup, vanilla and salt in a saucepan on a low heat until the cacao is completely dissolved into the liquid. It should resemble melted chocolate.

Add the almond butter and stir until thickened.

Spread over the cooled muffins.

Sweet potato brownies with macadamia-vanilla cream

These rich, decadent brownies are a seriously chocolate-y treat, but the sweetness comes from natural sources and the chocolate from raw cacao, which is higher in antioxidants and unlike a standard chocolate bar, doesn't contain any added dairy, soy lecithin or sugar. Sweet potatoes and ground almonds give these brownies a soft texture that's slightly squidgy in the middle, as all good brownies should be!

Ingredients
Makes 12 brownies

Brownies
1 large (or 2 smaller) sweet potatoes
1 cup ground almonds
¼ cup brown rice flour
10 tbsp. raw cacao powder
½ cup maple syrup/agave
2 flax eggs
1 tsp bicarb soda
1 tsp vanilla extract
pinch of sea salt

Macadamia cream
1 cup macadamias (or you could use cashews if you can't get macadamias) pre-soaked for 4 hours
3 tbsp. maple syrup
1 tbsp. lemon juice
1 tbsp. water
1 vanilla pod, deseeded
1 tsp coconut oil
pinch of sea salt

Make it

Preheat the oven to 375F/190C/Gas Mark 4. Line a brownie pan with baking paper.

Prepare the flax eggs – 1 tbsp. flax seed meal to 3 tbsp. water – and set aside for 10-15 mins

Bake the sweet potato in the microwave for around 7-10 mins, depending on size. Turn the potato half way through and remember to pierce several times with a fork before cooking.

Scoop out the flesh of the cooked sweet potato after it has cooled and discard the skin. Combine this in a bowl with the wet ingredients and mix well until it resembles a thick paste. You could use a stand mixer to do this if you have one.

Combine the dry ingredients in a separate bowl, then add them gradually to the sweet potato mixture, folding in as you add them.

Pour the mixture into the brownie pan and bake for 25-30 mins or until a skewer inserted into the center comes out clean.

Leave to cool.

Make the macadamia cream by adding all the ingredients to the blender and pulsing on high until you have a smooth texture with no chunks of nut left. If the mixture gets too thick and stops moving, you can add a little more water.

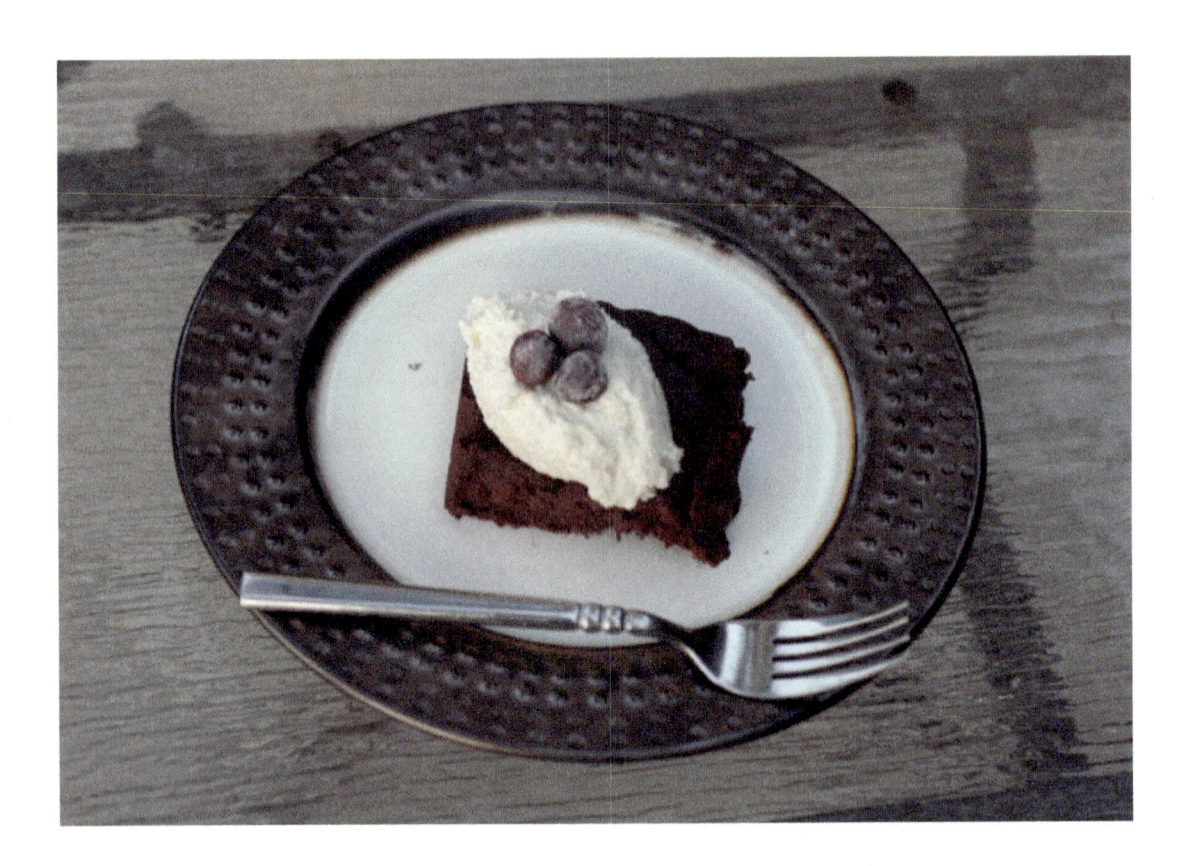

Banana zucchini bread

This is really a multi-purpose bake – it's good for a breakfast on the go or a snack, as it's high energy and also fiber-filled, which means it'll keep you satisfied, unlike a commercially made cake full of refined sugar and starch. This is one of Carly's mom Marilyn's favorites – and this lady knows her cakes.

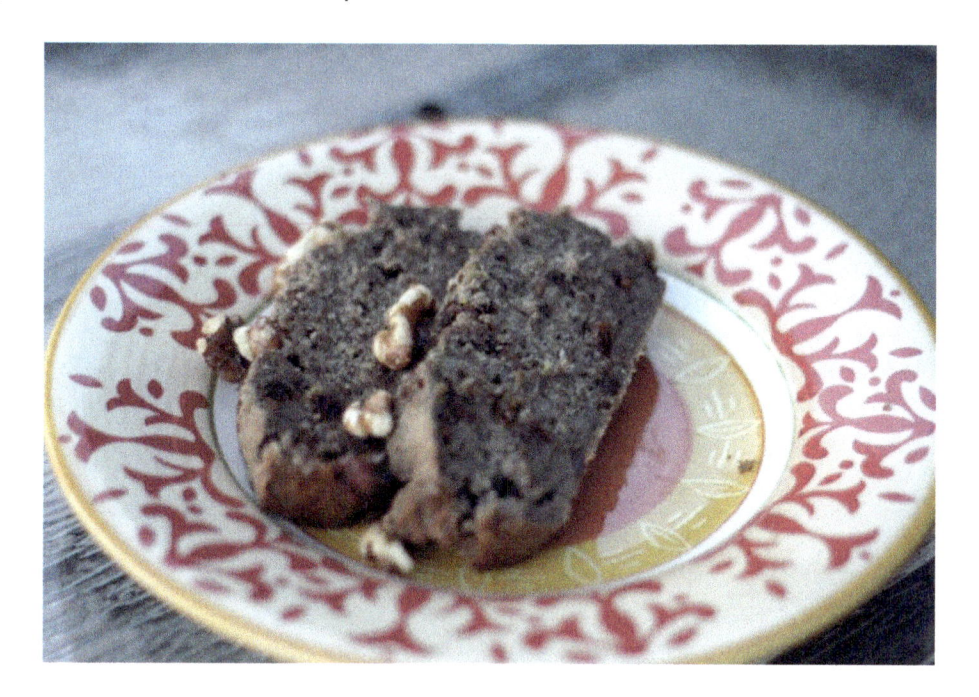

Ingredients
Makes 1 loaf in a 1lb loaf tin

2 ripe bananas, mashed
1 zucchini, finely shredded
1 cup buckwheat flour
1/2 cup brown rice flour
½ cup maple syrup/agave
1 cup raisins
1 flax egg
1 tsp vanilla extract
1 tsp bicarb soda
pinch of sea salt
A few walnut halves to decorate (optional)

Make it

Preheat the oven to 400F/200C/Gas Mark 5. Line a 1lb loaf tin with baking paper.

Make the flax egg – combine 1 tbsp. flaxseed meal with 3 tbsp. water. Set aside for 10-15 mins.

Mash the bananas and shred the zucchini. Add the flax egg, maple syrup and vanilla.

Combine the dry ingredients separately and then fold them into the wet ingredients a little at a time.

Stir through the raisins. Arrange the walnut halves on top if using, pushing them into the dough mix slightly so they stick well.

Pour into the loaf tin and spread evenly. Bake for around 40-45 mins, or until a skewer inserted into the middle comes out clean.

Juices and mocktails

Juicing is great for packing a whole lot of micronutrients into a small space. Vegetable juices are great for detoxing and cleansing your system. In this section, you'll find a few ideas for delicious combinations to get you started if you're new to juicing, You'll also find some ideas for non-alcoholic drinks to get you through the 'wine o'clock' temptation hour.

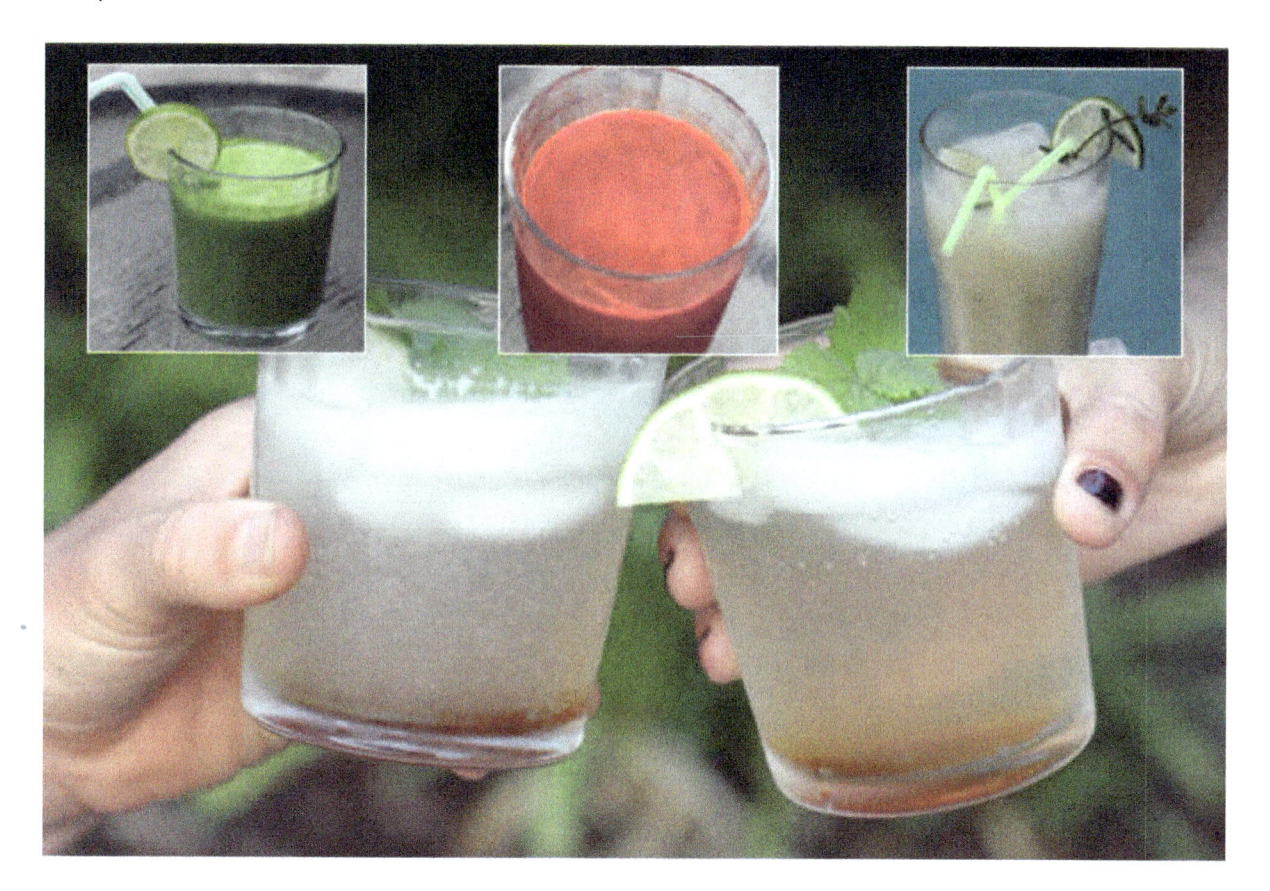

A note about alcohol
While alcohol isn't 'forbidden' on a whole food plant-based diet, we do advise not drinking frequently - save it for special occasions. Alcoholic drinks are basically empty calories, so they're not going to help if your goal is weight loss. Alcohol also dehydrates, leading to the dreaded hangover headache, along with bloating and water retention. It can also disrupt sleep and lead to low mood, so we advise caution. If you are going to drink, choose non-sugary drinks such as dry white wine or Prosecco, or clear spirits like gin and vodka with tonic or soda water and fresh lime.

Veggie power

You'll probably have seen vegetable juice in cans or bottles on the shelves at the grocery store. This freshly-juiced version is much healthier -- it's straight from the vegetables and not concentrated, so the nutrients will be alive and kicking! Spice this juice up with a little Tabasco sauce for a Virgin Mary-style juice experience.

Ingredients
Makes 4 200ml glasses

6-8 carrots
2 beets, plus tops
4-5 tomatoes
4 celery sticks
1 small cucumber (or ½ large one)
1 lemon
Pinch of sea salt and pepper
Few drops of Tabasco to serve, if desired

Juice it

Wash all the veggies thoroughly before juicing and peel the lemon, as the peel can make the juice too bitter.

Juice all the vegetables, add a little salt and pepper and stir. Pour into glasses and add a few drops of Tabasco sauce if you want some heat.

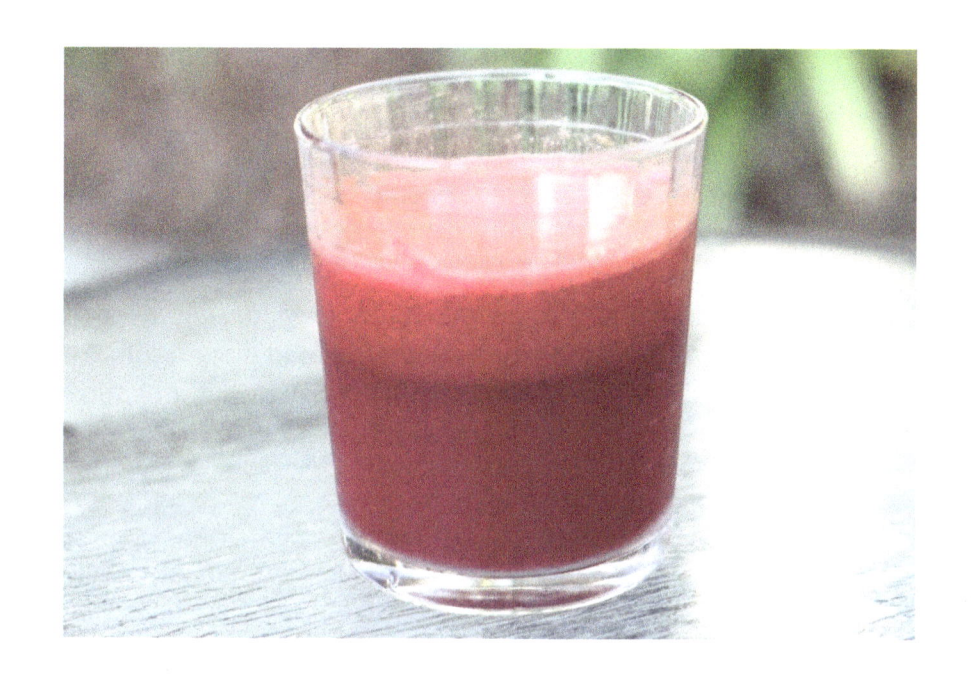

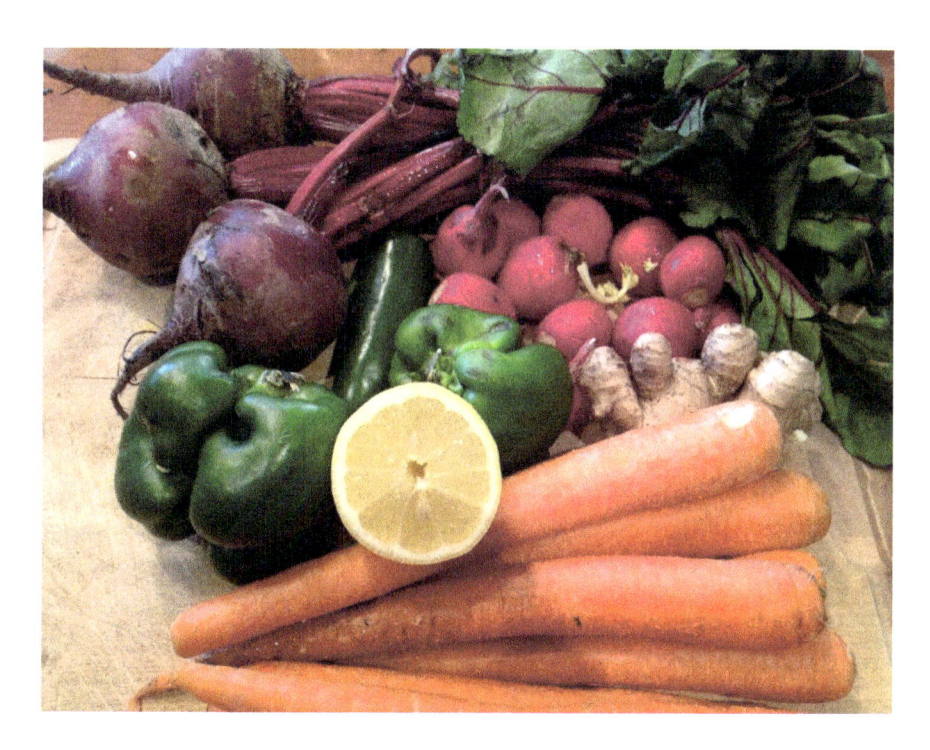

Mean green

Harness the power of green veggies and fruits with our "Mean Green" juice. Although all fruits and veggies are superfoods, green leafy vegetables like kale, spinach and chard are particular nutritional powerhouses– and yes, they contain protein too. Green leafy veggies contain chlorophyll, which is the substance that gives them their green color and allows them to absorb energy from sunlight. This is good for human health too, because it promotes healthy circulation and contains iron and magnesium. Furthermore, green leafy vegetables contain lots of Vitamin C and lutein, which is an antioxidant that protects against age-related eye problems such as cataracts and macular degeneration.

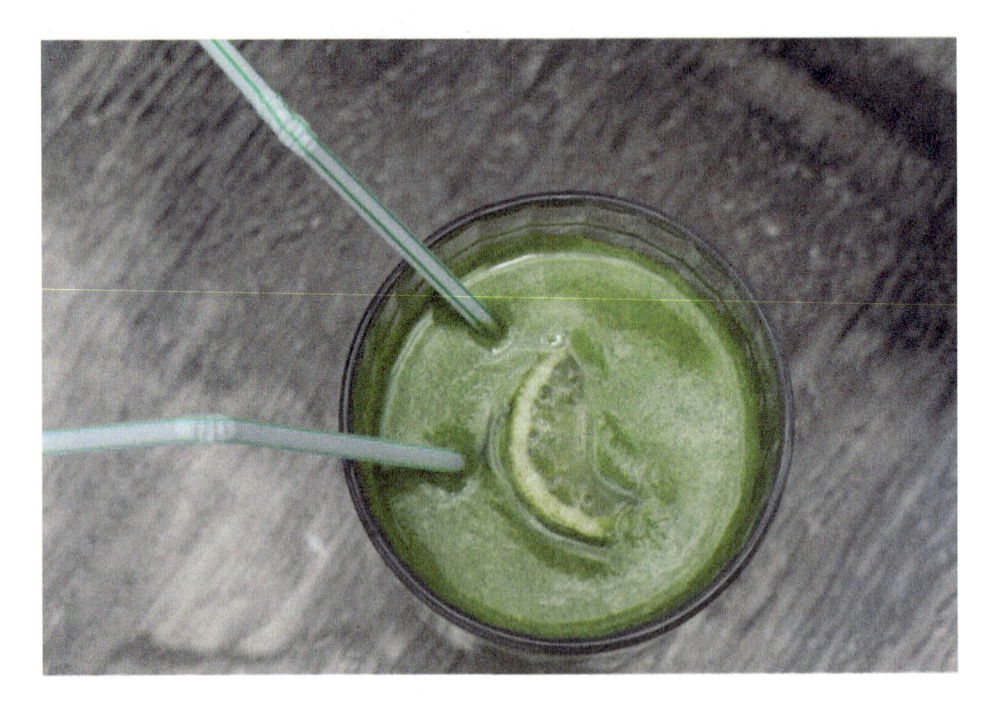

Ingredients
Makes 3-4x 200ml glasses

Handful of kale stems (you want whole stems for this, not the bags of shredded kale)
Handful of chard stems
2 generous handfuls of spinach leaves
1 head of romaine lettuce
1 small or ½ large cucumber
4 celery sticks
2 kiwi fruit
2 apples
1 lime

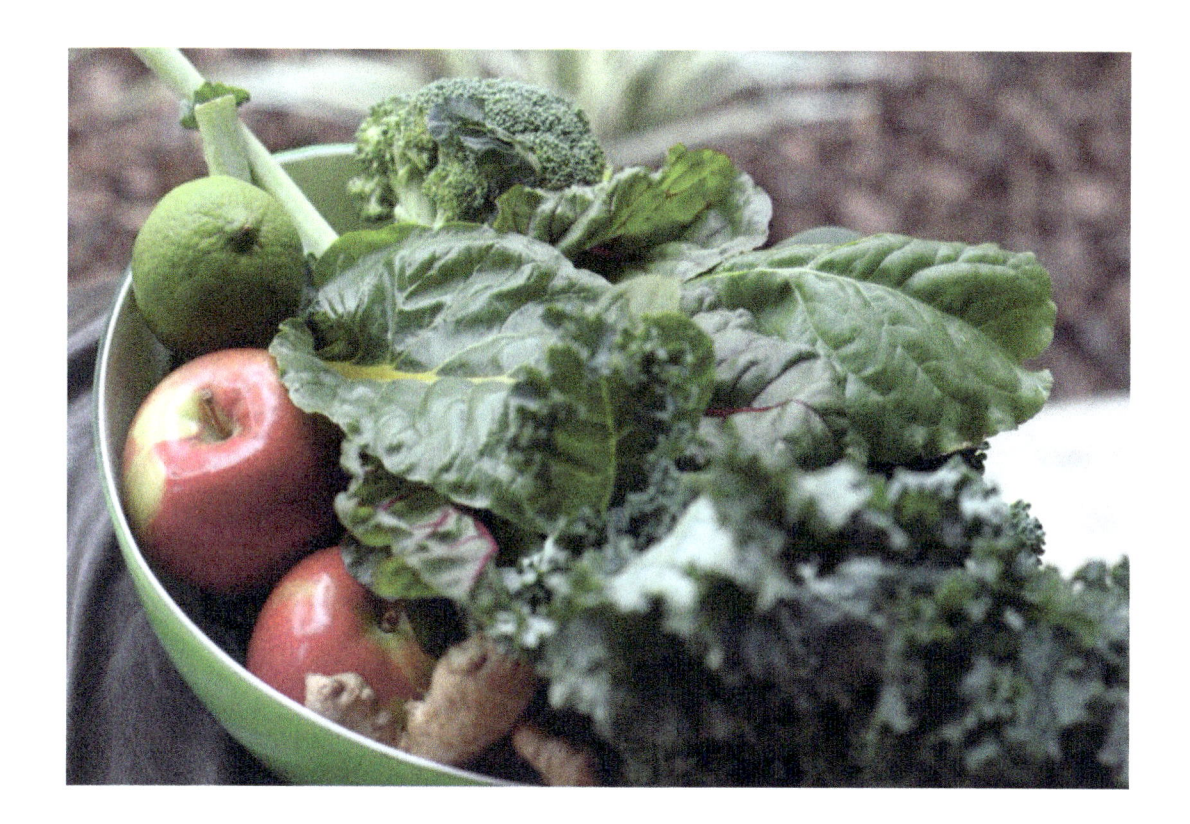

Make it

Wash your fruit and veg thoroughly. Peel the lime to avoid any bitterness in your juice.

Juice the fruits, cucumber and celery first. Feed the greens into the juicer a couple of stems at a time and push down well so they don't get stuck in the mechanism.

Give the juice a stir before serving.

Florida special

This juice is a fruity Vitamin C-packed cocktail straight from sunny tropical Florida, Carly's home state (and Liz's favorite escape from the British winter). These fruits are pretty easy to get hold of in a warm climate like Florida, but you may have to go hunting a little more if you live in a cooler place. Asian supermarkets are particularly good sources of tropical fruits and they will usually be cheaper than the regular supermarket too.

This juice makes particular use of citrus fruits and papaya. Citrus fruits are known for their high Vitamin C content and papaya contains an enzyme called papain, which is good for digestion and has been found to alleviate irritable bowel symptoms.

Ingredients
Makes 4x 200ml glasses

4-6 oranges (if they're large oranges, 4 should suffice, but you may need more if they're only small)
1 pink grapefruit
1 lemon
½ large orange papaya, deseeded
2 honey mangoes (or if you can't get honey mangoes, use 1 regular mango as they tend to be bigger)

Make it

Wash all fruits well before use.

Peel the citrus fruits and deseed the papaya. Cut the papaya into strips small enough to pass through your juicer.

Using a sharp knife, cut the flesh of the mangoes away from the stone. It's fine to leave the skin on as long as you've washed the mango well, but you can't juice the stone -- this will risk breaking your juicer.

Juice all ingredients and stir before serving.

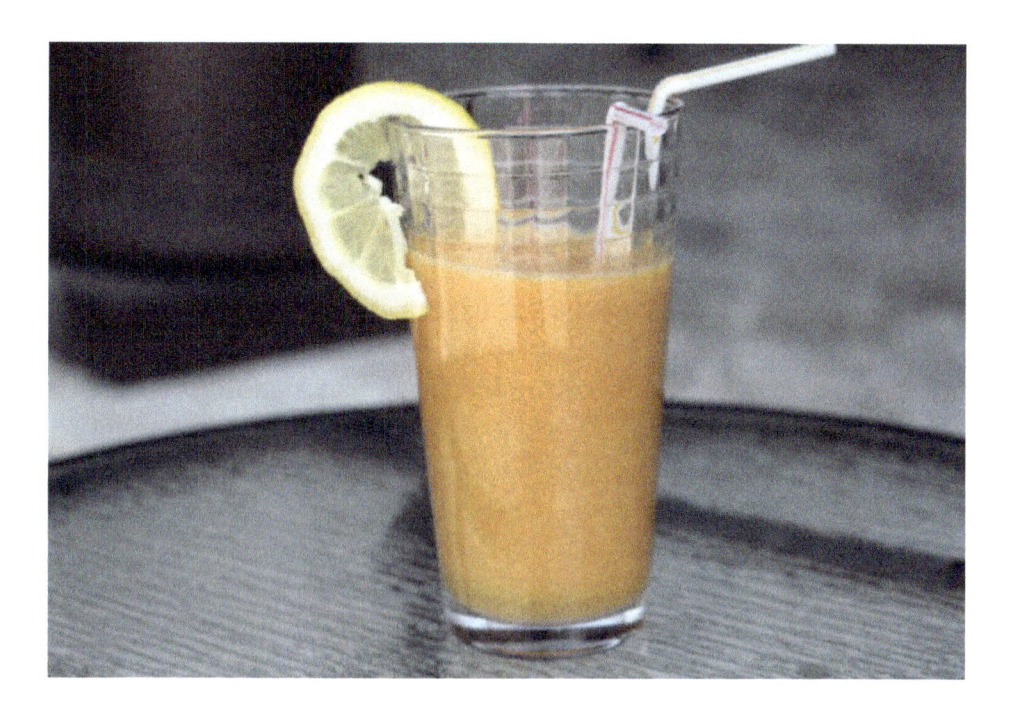

A note about fresh juices
Fresh juices are best drunk straight after juicing, as within a short space of time the live nutrients in the juice will start to deteriorate. If you want to store juice for later, the best way of doing this is to fill an airtight container to the top with the juice, store it in the fridge and drink it within a day. You can also freeze fresh juice, but do it straight after juicing, again, ensure the container is airtight and use the fast freeze compartment. Consume the frozen juice within 7-10 days.

Cold buster

This therapeutic juice is for keeping those winter bugs at bay. Citrus fruit and carrots provide Vitamin C, which is a good immune booster, while ginger is a traditional Asian remedy for colds and flu widely used in Chinese and Indian Ayurvedic medicine in particular. Ginger can also help relieve nausea and travel sickness. If your cold is making your chest or sinuses feel blocked, ginger has expectorant properties, which means it will help break down and release any congestion. Turmeric is a natural anti-inflammatory, which helps with pain, discomfort and inflammation. You can often buy fresh turmeric root in the supermarket, along with the fresh herbs and spices such as ginger and garlic, or in Asian grocery stores. If you can't find it, you could stir through 1 tsp turmeric powder at the end.

If the flavors in this juice are a little strong, you can add a teaspoon of agave to sweeten it a little.

Ingredients
Makes 3-4x 200ml glasses

4-6 oranges
4-6 carrots, preferably with the tops still attached
1 lemon
1 thumb sized piece of fresh ginger root
1 tbsp. fresh turmeric root (or 1tsp powder)

Make it

Wash everything well before use.

Peel the oranges and lemon.

Juice the carrots, ginger and turmeric root first, followed by the citrus fruits.

Stir the juice before serving – this is the time to stir through the turmeric powder, if you're using it.

Virgin mojito

This is a cool, refreshing long drink, perfect for serving at summer BBQs or as an alternative to your usual alcoholic pre-dinner drink. Another bonus is that this is much cheaper than the alcoholic version too, so you can slim your food and drink budget while you're UnSupersizing.

Ingredients
Makes 1 liter/4x 250ml glasses

Juice of 8 limes, plus a lime wedge or two for each glass to serve
4 tsp agave
Handful of mint leaves
Soda water/sparkling mineral water
Ice, either cubed or crushed, to serve

Make it

Half-fill your glasses with cubed or crushed ice.

Squeeze over the lime juice.

Drizzle 1 tsp agave in each glass.

Top up with sparkling water and mint and stir well to dissolve the agave.

Serve with extra wedges of lime.

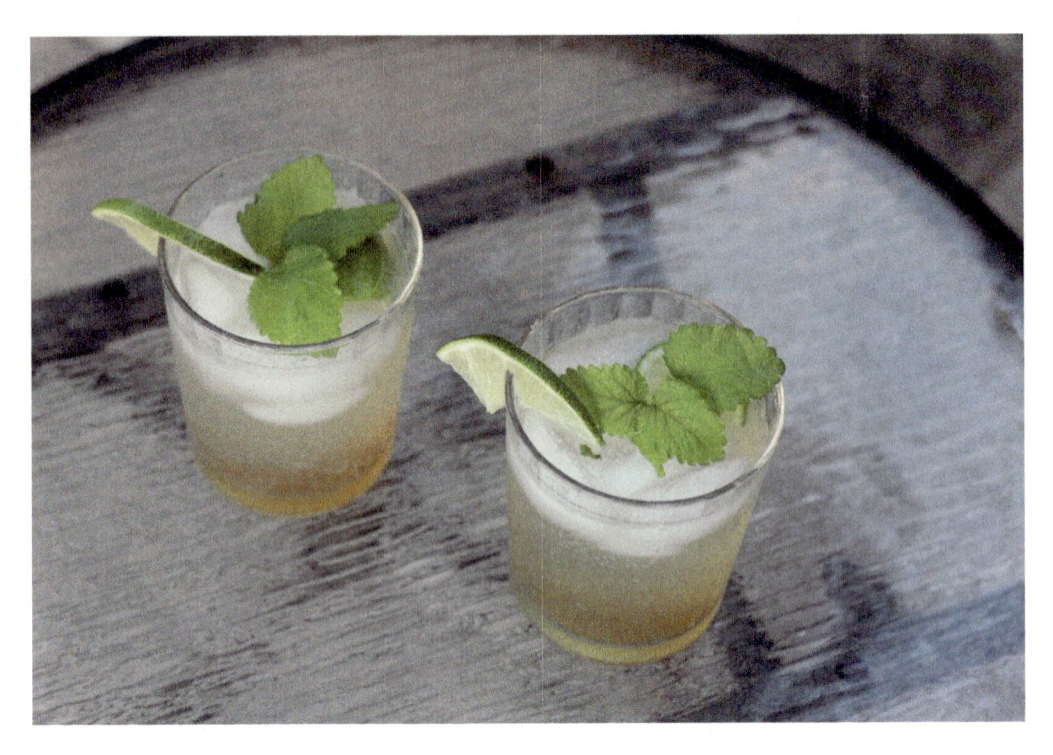

The Virgin Mojito

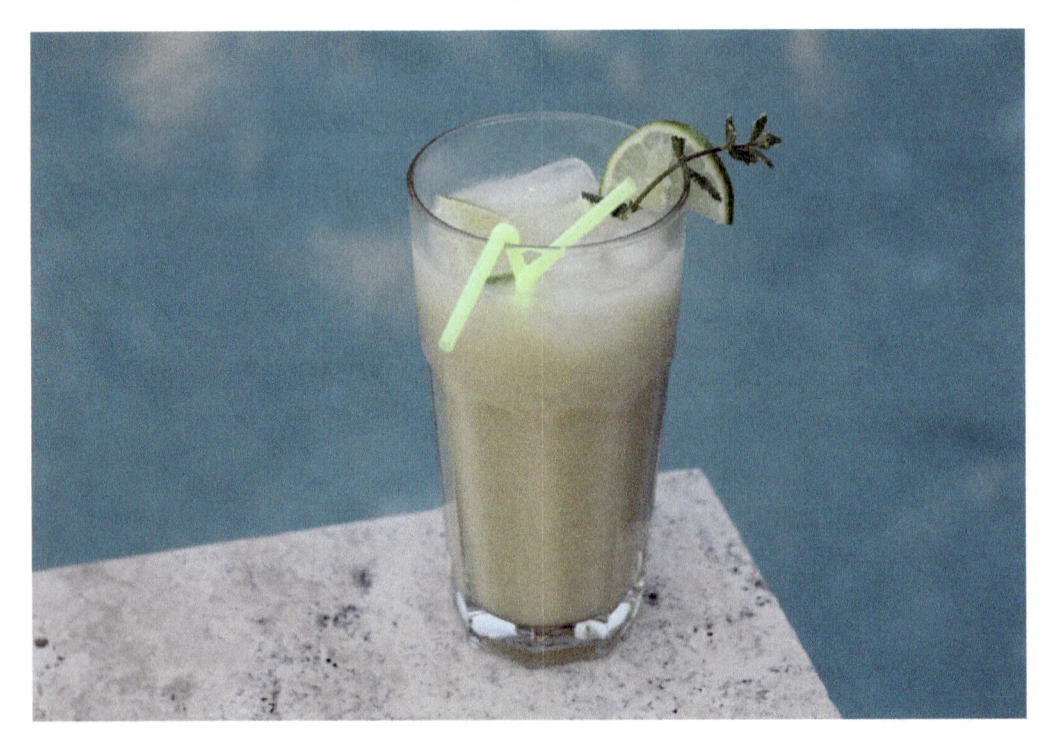

The non-alcoholic Piña Colada

Non-alcoholic Piña Colada

The tropical flavors of pineapple and coconut are combined in this mocktail, which is a fantastic summer treat. This is very simple to make too, but the luxurious creamy texture will no doubt impress your guests. Sharp lime will cut through the richness of the coconut milk.

Ingredients
Makes 1 liter/4x 250ml glasses

1 pineapple, skin removed and cut into wedges
2 cans light coconut milk
Juice of 2 limes
Ice and lime wedges to serve

Make it

Juice the fresh pineapple wedges in the juicer.

Pour the cans of coconut milk into a jug and stir well to ensure there is no separation or lumps.

Add the pineapple juice slowly to the coconut milk and stir to combine.

Stir through the lime juice. Add ice cubes to the glasses before pouring and serve with a wedge of lime in each glass.

Secret-weapon snacks

As *UnSupersize Us* subject Allison Ables always says, make like a Girl Scout and always be prepared. These snacks are great for eating on the run, before or after workouts. Some of them could be kept in your bag or car for emergency supplies. Being hungry when you're out and about and having nothing available to eat is a big danger zone that we want to avoid.

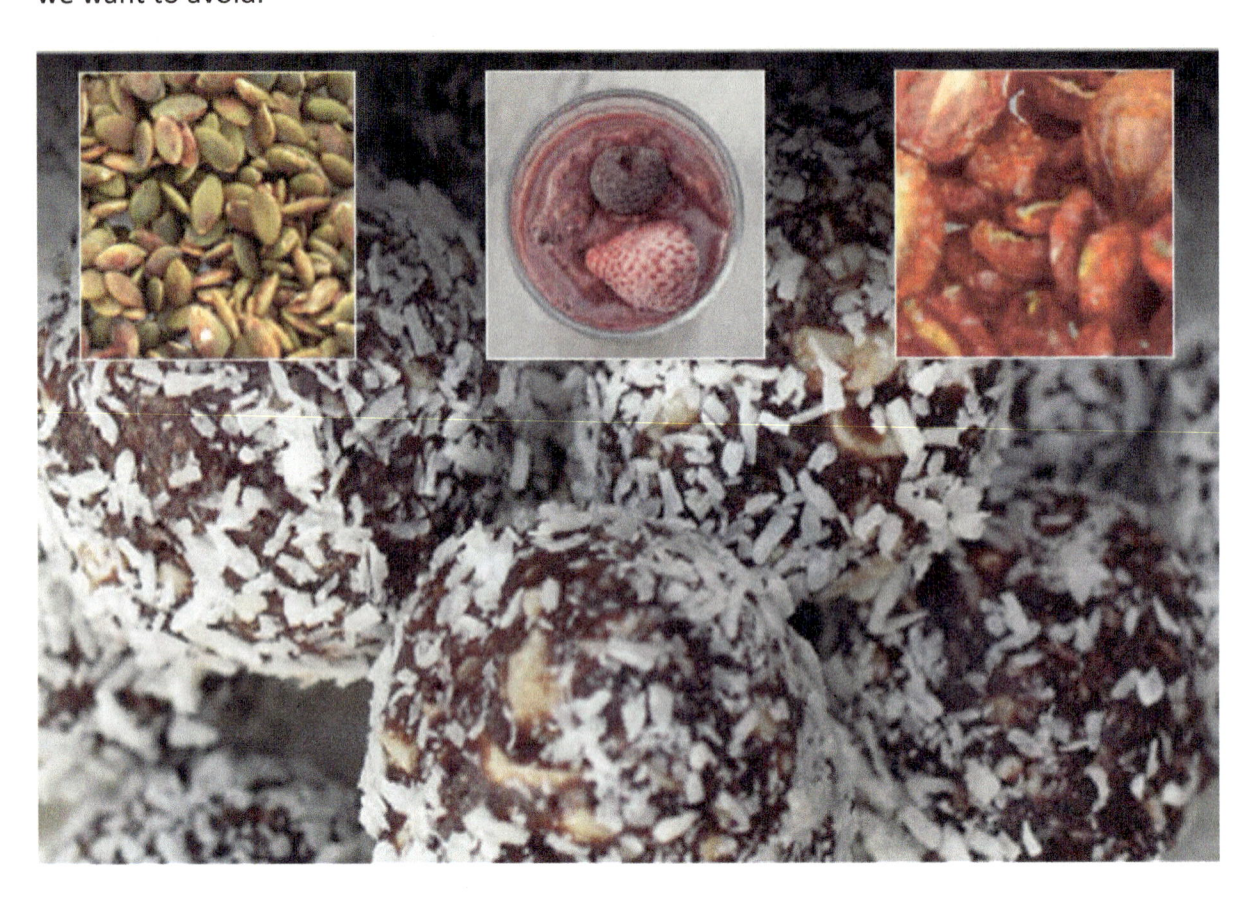

Sundried tomatoes

Yes, you can make these easily at home – no need to buy them in the supermarket in jars full of vegetable oil. They're so easy the recipe speaks for itself.

Ingredients

1 pack cherry or Roma plum tomatoes
1 tsp sea salt

Make it

Preheat the oven on a low heat – around 200F/70C/Gas Mark 1.

Wash, dry and halve the tomatoes.

Arrange the tomatoes on a baking sheet and sprinkle evenly with the salt.

Put them in the oven and allow to bake for around 2-2.5 hours. The tomatoes will dry out slowly, as they would in the traditional Italian sun-drying method, but this is obviously a bit quicker!

You can snack on these, add them to nuts and seeds to liven them up a bit, or use them in cooking or salads.

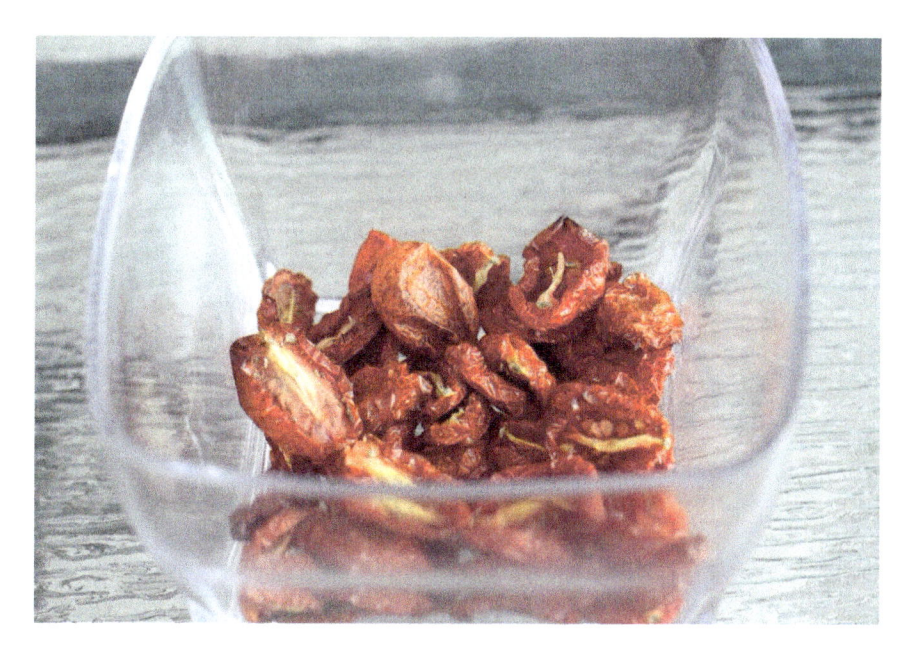

Tamari-roasted pumpkin seeds

This super simple recipe, using healthy fat-rich pumpkin seeds, could either be a snack food or a topping for salad or stir fry. These also keep well in an airtight container, are portable and don't need to be refrigerated.

Ingredients

1 cup shelled raw pumpkin seeds (pepitas)
2 tbsp. soy sauce/gluten free tamari

Make it

Heat a frying pan/skillet to high temperature.

Drop the pumpkin seeds in and spread evenly over the pan surface.

Dry roast them in the pan, stirring to ensure they don't burn on the bottom.

You will start to hear them make a popping sound as they roast. When this happens, remove from the heat and add the tamari and coat the seeds evenly.

Leave to cool and then store in an airtight container.

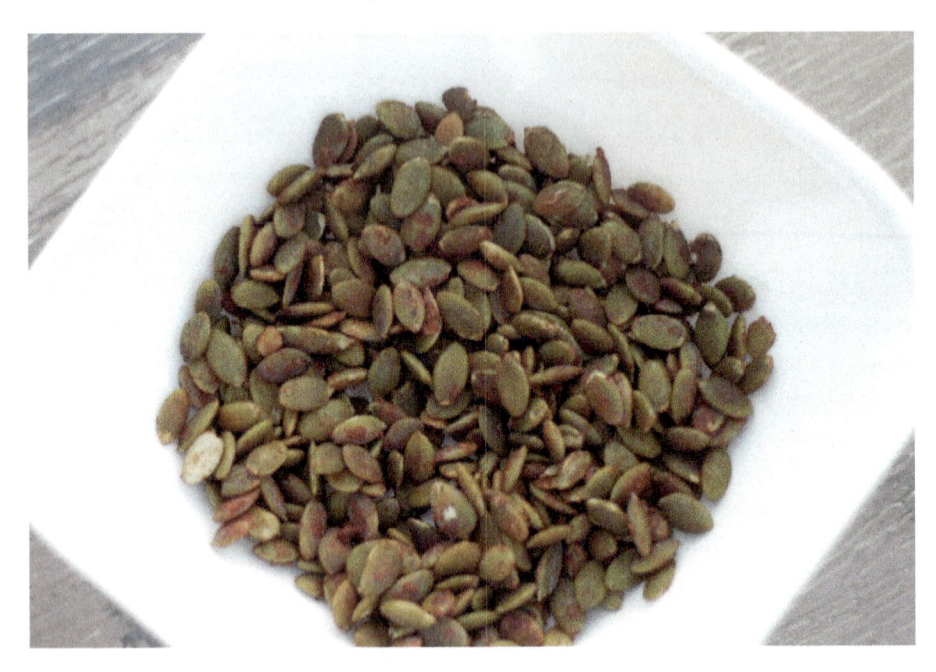

Chia berry jam

This is a recipe that Liz came up with because she was missing good old English jam. Jam (or jelly) might be made from fruit, but it's not a food that we recommend on a whole food plant based diet, because commercial jams have sugar, high fructose corn syrup, thickeners and gums, and often artificial sweeteners too – yuck!

Chia seeds offer the jam enthusiast a perfect solution, because they absorb liquid and can be used to thicken. This jam is quick to make, spreads well and will keep in the fridge.

Ingredients
Makes 2 large jars

3 cups berries (if you use frozen berries allow them to defrost first)
1 cup water
Juice of 1/2 lemon
1/2 cup natural sweetener such as agave, date syrup or maple syrup (agave doesn't have too much of a distinct flavor and allows the flavor of the berries to come through)
1/3 cup chia seeds

Make it

Put the berries, water and sweetener in a saucepan and bring slowly to the boil.

Once it comes just to boiling point, turn down to a simmer and leave for around 15-20 mins until everything is combined and the berries start to break down a little. Berries such as raspberries, blackberries, blackcurrants and redcurrants will break down more quickly than blueberries or cherries, so depending on whether you like to still have a little texture in your jam, you may wish to simmer them for longer if you prefer not to have chunks of fruit in there.

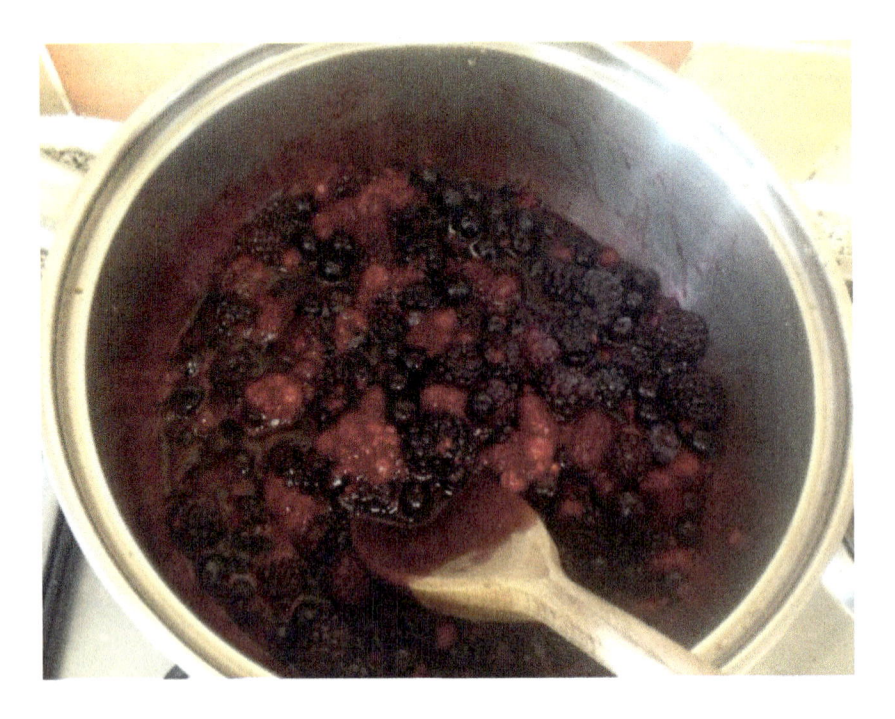

Add the chia seeds, stirring as you add them. Remove from the heat and mix the seeds in well, ensuring they are coated in the mixture. If it seems like they're not getting fully coated, you can add more water. The water content of the mixture may vary a little depending on what kinds of berries you use.

The chia seeds will take around 15 mins to absorb the excess water and give it that slightly gloopy, jammy texture.

Pour into sterilized containers. This is also a great way to recycle jars, since we hate wasting anything around here!

If you want to use old jars, you'll need to wash them (and their lids) in hot soapy water first, rinse them well, then put them into a preheated oven set to 140C (120 fan)/Gas 1. They should be heated in the oven until they are completely dry. If you have Kilner/mason jars, the method is the same, but don't put the rubber seals in the oven - sterilize them in boiling water instead. Put a waxed or greaseproof paper disc on top of the jam when you have filled the jar to keep the air from getting to it.

Keep your jam refrigerated.

Once opened, we recommend using it within 2 weeks.

Cherry-strawberry-chocolate smoothie

Smoothies make a great snack on the go. They're quick to make and a great use for frozen fruit, so you know your smoothie will be nice and chilled. This smoothie, which is one of Carly's favorites, is almost like a blended Black Forest gateau, but a lot healthier and without all that dairy. Get yourself a portable smoothie cup so you can take your smoothies to work or for a post-workout energy boost.

Ingredients
Serves 2

1/2 cup frozen strawberries
1/2 cup frozen cherries
1 tbsp. cacao powder
5 medjool dates
1 cup vanilla cashew milk (or other dairy free milk of your choice)

Simply blend and enjoy!

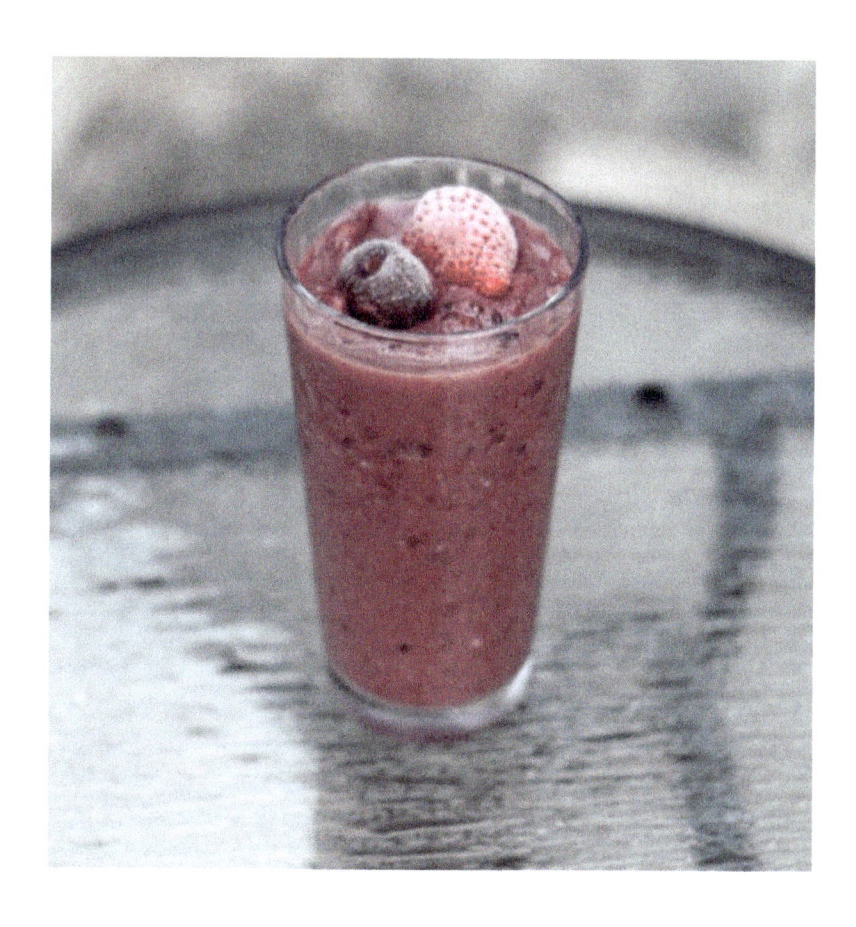

Healthy cacao-date 'truffles'

These cute little balls of chocolate-y goodness don't look like they'd be good for you, but we assure you they are! They are made from raw cacao, so you'll get your daily dose of flavones, the antioxidants found in the cacao bean. Flavones have been shown to help protect against age-related cognitive decline, so using raw cacao is a healthy way to get them in your diet. These could be a healthy snack or an after dinner treat.

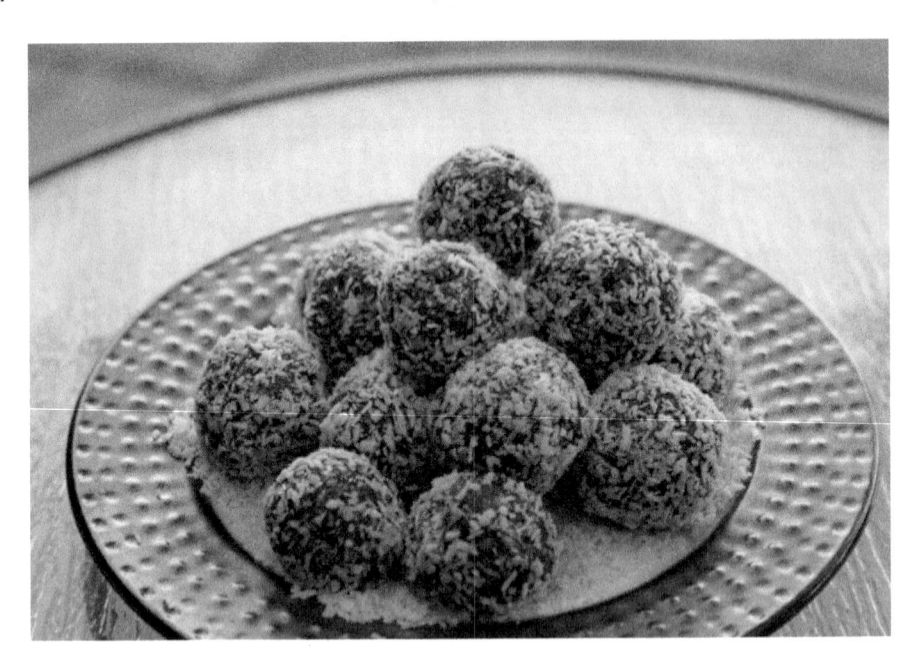

Ingredients
Makes 12 truffles

12 medjool dates, pitted
4 tbsp. raw cacao
2 tbsp. coconut oil
½ cup cashews, soaked in cold water for 4 hrs.
2 tbsp. flaxseed meal
1 tsp vanilla extract
4 tbsp. maple syrup or agave
Shredded coconut, for decoration

Make it

Roughly chop the cashews and dates.

Place the ingredients in a high-speed heavy duty blender.

Pulse to combine ingredients. The mixture can get a little sticky, so if it does, you can add a little water to loosen it so it blends.

Coat the base of a plate with shredded coconut. Roll into individual balls, then roll in the coconut.

Chill in the refrigerator for an hour before serving. Store in an airtight container.

If you want to transport these, it's important to place them in a Pyrex or BPA-free food storage container, because if they are put in a plastic bag they will quickly start to "sweat" and melt.

More Resources

If you loved this book and want to know more about anything you've read here, you can go to the **UnSupersize Me website,** http://unsupersizeme.com and check out the films, our bookstore, and the options available for doing the UnSupersize Me program for yourself.

For information about training at **Zen Fitness** in Gainesville, visit
http://www.thezenfitness.com/

Contact us and follow us on social media!

Find UnSupersize Me on Facebook: https://www.facebook.com/unsupersizeme/
Tweet UnSupersize Me: @UnSupersize_Me
Connect with us on Instagram: @UnSupersizeMe
Email Carly: carly@thezenfitness.com
Email Liz: wordscene@gmail.com

Other places for helpful information on the whole food plant-based diet, weight loss and fitness:

Clean Food Dirty Girl – nutrition coaching, whole food plant-based recipes, whole food plant-based Facebook group and more.
http://cleanfooddirtygirl.com/

PlantPure Nation – Film, information about local plant-based groups, recipe books and diet resources.
http://www.plantpurenation.com/

Forks Over Knives – Film, recipes (and book available), nutrition help and coaching and diet resources.
http://www.forksoverknives.com/

No Meat Athlete – Matt Frazier, the No Meat Athlete, provides resources for vegan and plant-based runners and other fitness fans. No Meat Athlete Radio has interesting podcasts with prominent vegan athletes and discussions on topics around fitness on a plant-based diet.
http://www.nomeatathlete.com/

©2016, Carly Asse and Liz Smith, all rights reserved

CPSIA information can be obtained
at www.ICGtesting.com
Printed in the USA
LVOW05s1044290816
502243LV00001B/1/P